Intermittent Fasting for Women over 50

A Scientific Plan to Accelerate Weight Loss, Increase Your Energy, and Improve your Health. Burn Fat and Feel Better without Sacrificing Your Favorite Foods

Clara Johnson

Table of Contents

INTRODUCTION

Intermittent fasting is an action of fasting intermittently. It is an eating pattern where you cycle between periods of eating and periods of voluntary fasting over a single day, week or other defined period. In layman's terms, it merely means controlling when you eat and when you don't. The period when you don't consume any food or drinks (besides water) is called a fasting window. And the rest is called...the eating window. How long you choose to make your fasting or eating window is really up to you and your chosen Intermittent Fasting schedule.

Intermittent fasting as the name implies, is fasting for a certain period, such as from 12 to 48 hours. The span is called 'fasting window', wherein you are allowed to drink bone broth, coffee, herbal tea, and water. It is recommended to take vitamins and consume juices made from low-calorie vegetables during the fasting periods as this keeps the mineral and vitamin levels consistent.

After the fasting window, an eating window follows. The common span for this window is 6 to 12 hours. The fasting and eating windows can vary as there are different IF methods, some being more intense than others. You can experiment between them, so you can find out which method suits you and your lifestyle the best.

Intermittent fasting for women can be very beneficial if done right. If calories are restricted too harshly, it may trigger an imbalance in hormones leading to issues like infertility and irregular periods.

Intermittent fasting has taken the Internet by storm. You see people sharing their journey of intermittent fasting on YouTube, while at the same time, some people think intermittent fasting is dumb. All kinds of debates have been going on about its practicality and effectiveness over the past few years. There is research that proves everything from the benefits of weight loss to promoting longevity, yet there are people who claim intermittent fasting is just another diet trend without sufficient evidence and proof on its benefits.

Thus, women who chose to do intermittent fasting should pay attention to the nutritional value of their diet. Otherwise, they can lose the benefits of IF and bring more harm than good to their bodies. A few things that make it tougher to lose weight after age 50 include lower metabolism, achy joints, reduced muscle mass, and even sleep issues. At the same time, losing fat, especially dangerous belly fat, can dramatically reduce your risk for such serious health issues as diabetes, heart attacks, and cancer.

Of course, as you age, the risk of developing many diseases increases. In some cases, intermittent fasting for women over 50 could serve as a virtual fountain of youth when it comes to weight loss and minimizing the chance of developing typically age-related illnesses.

Women over 50 usually undergo the pre and post-menopausal stages and the fat accumulation in their midsection increases. Belly fat is not only the hardest fat to lose, but is also associated with plenty of risks such as type II diabetes, higher blood pressure and high levels of cholesterol. To avoid such issues intermittent fasting is an ideal way to keep you fit and healthy.

Several studies indicate that IF is especially effective in reducing belly fat. This is attributed to the increased production of human growth hormone, which helps the body to burn fat. The HGH levels increase when insulin is low. So, when you combine intermittent fasting with good sleep and effective exercise, the resultant low insulin helps boost the HGH and increases fat burning.

CHAPTER 1: INTERMITTENT FASTING

Intermittent fasting involves alternating periods of feast and famine in which you may eat as much as you like during the feasting, but drink only water during the fast. The aim is to achieve the benefits of calorie reduction and for some, use it as a vehicle to lose weight. Intermittent fasting can be done over some days, in alternating 24 hour periods or daily.

The first option requires you abstain from some or all meals on one or more days of the week. Daily fasting utilizes 24 hour periods of eating and fasting that begin and end at the same time each day, for example, fast from Monday 6 pm until Tuesday 6 pm, eat as much as you like from Tuesday 6 pm to Wednesday at 6 pm and repeat the process. During daily intermittent fasting there is a short period for eating, usually, 4-6 hours within the 24 hour day during which you can eat as much as you like.

Some of the things that put people off are the fear they will be extremely hungry and not stick to the plan or do not know how to fit it into their schedule. This is quite simple if you plan. You get to eat your evening meal at pretty much the same time every day, but at an hour either side depending on if you are in an intermittent fasting phase or an eating phase. Again with a little planning you can also accommodate socializing and eating out.

Intermittent fasting has become quite a phenomenon these days. Recent studies showed people who have tried it have lost weight, increased health, and are believed to have a long lifespan. Intermittent fasting is a pattern of eating that alternates between periods of fasting, usually consuming only water, and non-fasting, usually eating anything a person wants no matter how fattening. In other words, a person can eat anything he wants during 24 hours and fast for the next 24 hours.

This approach to weight control seems to be supported by science, as well as religious and cultural practices around the globe. Adherents of intermittent fasting claim this practice is a way to become more circumspect about food. There are many different popular intermittent fasts and hundreds of more possible variations. There are two kinds of intermittent fasts that are the most basic and frequently used.

- First is the daily fasting in which the person only gets to eat once every 20-28 hours within 4 hours.
- The second is fasting for 1-3x a week, also called alternate day fasting, in which a person eats anything he wants on one day and fasts the whole of the next day.

Intermittent fasting has many beneficial effects as tested on animals like rodents and primates. One study found that there has been a "reduced serum glucose and insulin levels and increased resistance of neurons in the brain to excitotoxic stress." In 2008, a study on intermittent fasting showed lifespan increases of 40.4% and 56.6% in C. elegans for an alternate day (24 hours) and two-of-each-three days (48 hours) fasting, respectively, as compared to an ad libitum diet.

What Is Intermittent Fasting (If)?

Fasting or periods of voluntary abstinence from food has been practiced throughout the world for ages. Intermittent fasting to improve health is relatively new. Intermittent fasting involves restricting the intake of food for a set period and does not include any changes to the actual foods you are eating. Currently, the most common IF protocols are a daily 16 hour fast and fasting for a whole day, one or two days per week. Intermittent fasting could be considered a natural eating pattern that humans are built to implement and it traces back to our paleolithic hunter-gatherer ancestors.

The current model of a planned program of intermittent fasting could potentially help improve many aspects of health from body composition to longevity and aging. Although IF goes against the norms of our culture and common daily routine, the science may be pointing to less meal frequency and more time fasting as the optimal alternative to the normal breakfast, lunch, and dinner model.

Intermittent Fasting?

It is an eating pattern where one fasts for a set period and then eats for another set period. The three most common approaches I have seen in the literature are the once a week/month, 24 hours and the daily 16/8 or 20/4 intermittent fast. During the 24 hour routine, the individual doesn't eat or drink anything except water, green tea and maybe some Branch Chain Amino Acids (BCAA) for 24 hours. Then, after that 24 hour period has expired they begin eating again. During the 16/8 or 20/4 routine, the individual does not eat for either 16 to 20 hours and then eats meals during the other 4 to 8 hour period.

Intermittent Fasting For Women Over 50

Our bodies and our metabolism changes when we hit menopause. One of the biggest changes women over 50 experience is they have a slower metabolism and they start to put on weight. Fasting may be a good way to reverse and prevent this weight gain though. Studies have shown this fasting pattern helps to regulate appetite and people who follow it regularly do not experience the same cravings that others do. If you're over 50 and trying to adjust to your slower metabolism, intermittent fasting can help you to avoid eating too much daily.

When you reach 50, your body also starts to develop some chronic diseases like high cholesterol and high blood pressure. Intermittent fasting has been shown to decrease both cholesterol and blood pressure, even without a great deal of weight loss. If you've started to notice your numbers rising at the doctor's office each year, you may be able to bring them back down with fasting, even without losing much weight.

Intermittent fasting may not be a great idea for every woman. Anyone with a specific health condition or who tends to be hypoglycemic should consult with a doctor. However, this new dietary trend has specific benefits for women who naturally store more fat in their bodies and may have trouble getting rid of these fat stores. Weight loss for women older than 50 isn't easy, but it's not impossible either. It takes dedication, smart food choices, and a commitment to staying active.

i. Learn To Enjoy Strength Training

Although cardio gets a lot of attention when it comes to weight loss, strength training is also important, especially for older adults. As you age, your muscle mass declines in a process called sarcopenia. This loss of muscle mass begins around the age of 50 and can slow your metabolism, which may lead to weight gain. After the age of 50, your muscle mass decreases by about 1–2% per year, while your muscle strength declines at a rate of 1.5–5% per year. Thus, adding muscle-building exercises to your routine is essential for reducing age-related muscle loss and promoting a healthy body weight.

Strength training, such as body weight exercises and weightlifting, can significantly improve muscle strength and increase muscle size and function Plus, strength training can help you lose weight by reducing body fat and boosting your metabolism, which can increase how many calories you burn throughout the day.

ii. Talk To Your Doctor About A Weight-Loss Plan

It's never a good idea to create a weight-loss plan for yourself without speaking to your physician first, especially if you have any preexisting health conditions. "Before you get started, it helps to fully understand your current state of health before beginning any diet or exercise plan." Be clear with your doctor about what you hope to achieve, and ask for suggestions regarding diet and exercise. Your doctor may even be able to recommend a physical therapist or personal trainer for you.

iii. Team Up

Introducing a healthy eating pattern or exercise routine on your own can be challenging. Pairing up with a friend, co-worker, or family member may give you a better chance at sticking to your plan and achieving your wellness goals. For example, research shows those who attend weight loss programs with friends are significantly more likely to maintain their weight loss over time. Additionally, working out with friends can strengthen your commitment to a fitness program and make exercising more enjoyable.

iv. Get Your Stress In Check

The average 50-year-old has many more responsibilities than their younger peers. They're often in their prime income-generating years, which means extra responsibilities at work. They may also have kids who are going to college, a financial burden or have aging parents who they're helping to care for."

The result? Emotional eating and a schedule that seems too jam-packed for regular exercise sessions. The solution: Schedule your workouts like they're doctor's appointments, Sticking to a consistent routine can not only help ease stress, but also help people stay on track with their diets. After all, who wants to ruin the benefits of a tough sweat session by eating a donut?

v. Sit Less And Move More

Burning more calories than you take in is critical to losing excess body fat. That's why being more active throughout the day is important when trying to lose weight. For example, sitting at your job for long periods might impede your weight loss efforts. To counteract this, you can become more active at work by simply getting up from your desk and taking a five-minute walk every hour.

Research shows that tracking your steps using a pedometer or Fitbit can boost weight loss by increasing your activity levels and calorie expenditure. When using a pedometer or Fitbit, start with a realistic step goal based on your current activity levels. Then gradually work your way up to 7,000–10,000 steps per day or more, depending on your overall health.

vi. Talk To A dietitian

Finding an eating pattern that both promotes weight loss and nourishes your body can be difficult. Consulting a registered dietitian can help you determine the best way to lose excess body fat without having to follow an overly restrictive diet. Also, a dietitian can support and guide you throughout your weight loss journey. Research shows that working with a dietitian to lose weight can lead to significantly better results than going at it alone, and it may help you maintain weight loss over time.

vii. Bump Up Your Protein Intake

Getting enough high-quality protein in your diet is not only important for weight loss but also critical for stopping or reversing age-related muscle loss. How many calories you burn at rest, or your resting metabolic rate (RMR), decreases by 1–2% each decade after you turn 20. This is associated with age-related muscle loss. However, eating a protein-rich diet can help prevent or even reverse muscle loss. Numerous studies have also shown that increasing dietary protein can help you lose weight and keep it off in the long term.

viii. Eat More Produce

Vegetables and fruits are packed with nutrients that are vital to your health, and adding them into your diet is a simple, evidence-based way to drop excess weight.For example, a review of 10 studies found that every daily serving increase of vegetables was associated with a 0.14-inch (0.36-cm) waist circumference reduction in women. Another study in women aged 35–65 associated eating fruits and vegetables with lower body weight, reduced waist circumference, and less body fat

ix. Rely less On Convenience Foods

Regularly eating convenience foods, such as fast food, candy, and processed snacks are associated with weight gain and may hinder your weight loss efforts. Convenience foods are typically high in calories and tend to be low in important nutrients like protein, fiber, vitamins, and minerals. That's why fast food and other processed foods are commonly referred to as "empty calories."Cutting back on convenience foods and replacing them with nutritious meals and snacks that revolve around nutrient-dense whole foods is a smart way to lose weight

x. Consume Adequate Protein

Protein is important for weight loss, as the macronutrient lends great satiety and regulates hunger hormones. It also curbs blood sugar fluctuation and supplies metabolic-supporting B vitamins. Protein is also essential in preserving muscle mass and strength. Current protein recommendations suggest adults 19 or older should eat 0.8 grams of protein per kilogram of body weight (g/kg).

However, growing research suggests adults aged 65 plus may require between 1.0 and 1.2 g/kg of protein daily. Those with sarcopenia, or muscle loss, may need 1.2 to 1.5 g/kg. Consult with a healthcare professional to assist in determining protein needs, too. This especially serves true if managing a health condition, such as kidney disease, as protein needs can vary. Consume lean and plant-based proteins to reduce overall calorie and fat intake fat. Sirloin, chicken, turkey, fish, eggs, beans, lentils, and other legumes are great sources of protein to include in a balanced diet.

xi. Eat Less At Night

Many studies have shown that eating fewer calories at night may help you maintain a healthy body weight and lose excess body fat. A study in 1,245 people found that over 6 years, those who consumed more calories at dinner were over 2 times more likely to become obese than people who ate more calories earlier in the day. Plus, those who ate more calories at dinner were significantly more likely to develop metabolic syndrome, a group of conditions including high blood sugar and excess belly fat.

Metabolic syndrome increases your risk of heart disease, diabetes, and stroke. Eating the majority of your calories during breakfast and lunch, while enjoying a lighter dinner, maybe a worthwhile method to promote weight loss.

xii. Strategize Fluid Needs

While good hydration is essential throughout the entire lifespan, growing older heightens the risk of dehydration. This is likely is related to a decreased thirst mechanism. Thirst often masks itself as hunger as well, which can direct attention to food rather than a glass of water. Hydration can also be in the form of foods that are naturally rich in water, including watermelon, celery, and cucumber.

But try to limit foods and drinks filled with empty calories, including soft drinks, energy drinks, and alcoholic beverages. And if you are to drink, men are advised to limit alcohol consumption to no more than two drinks per day. Women are encouraged to drink 11.5 cups (2.7 liters) of fluids daily.

xiii. Try Out Intermittent Fasting

Intermittent fasting is a type of eating pattern in which you only eat during a specified period. The most popular type of intermittent fasting is the 16/8 method, where you eat within an 8-hour window followed by a 16-hour fast). Numerous studies have shown that intermittent fasting promotes weight loss. What's more, some test-tube and animal studies suggest intermittent fasting may benefit older adults by increasing longevity, slowing cell decline, and preventing age-related changes to mitochondria, the energy-producing parts of your cells.

xiv. Say "No" To Sugary Drinks

You've heard it before and I'll say it again, drinks like energy drinks, fruit juices, and that beloved soda is loaded with sugars and unnecessary calories that only add to the weight you're trying to lose. Sugary drinks are simply empty calories. They lack any nutritional benefits and don't fill you up but still add to your daily calorie count. Thanks to the added sugars, such drinks also make you more prone to storing body fat–especially around your midsection.

On top of that, the most popular sugary drink of all, soda, harms more than just the number on the scale. It also negatively effects your:

- Heart
- Brain
- Bones
- Teeth

Why risk your health so drastically when you could simply swap out sugary drinks, like soda, for water? You could live a much healthier life and take steps closer to reaching your goal weight by making this simple change. This may be the easiest and most beneficial of these best weight loss tips for women over 50!

xv. Balance Your Workouts.

It's great if you do any exercise daily. But as we age, a balanced workout program becomes more important. a varied program can offset hormonal and body composition changes that happen as we get older. Make sure your program includes these elements.

- Strength Training: Do resistance or strength training exercises to build and maintain muscle and to keep your metabolism healthy. Studies have shown that resistance (strength) training has specific benefits for us as we age.
- Aerobic training: Do cardiovascular activity regularly to offset the decrease in metabolism that comes with age and to improve your heart health.
- Flexibility training: Do stretching exercises to increase the range of motion in your joints. This helps your body stay limber and comfortable through activities of daily living.

What Makes Intermittent Fasting Different?

Intermittent fasting weight loss is one of the most effective ways to shed off your extra pounds. The ideas on intermittent fasting weight loss challenge most of the previously held beliefs on losing. Those who are seeking new ways to lose weight effectively have quickly embraced their ideas.

What is Intermittent Fasting Weight Loss?

Let me start by clarifying that intermittent fasting is not a diet. You are probably tired of trying anything with the word 'diet' on it when it comes to weight loss. Intermittent fasting is a way of eating that involves a structured program on the times when you eat and when you do not eat. You structure your program according to your fancy. If you can handle it, fast for a whole day! I recommend that you fast for 12 full hours before eating a meal. You can increase your fasting period later as you continue with the program.

What Makes It Different?

If you have tried to lose weight, you probably have tried diets such as the Atkins diet based on the frequent feeding theory. Simply, proponents of such diets told you to eat often during the day. The idea was that the more you eat, the faster your metabolism. The faster your metabolism, the more fat you will lose. Of course, you do know that the more you ate, the more you wanted to eat and the more your weight remained. When you are on an intermittent fasting program, you will have to cut down your meal frequency. Sometimes, you have to do without breakfast.

Tell Me More

You probably sleep for around 6 to 8 hours. During this time, your body is in fasting mode. When your body is in fasting mode, it usually produces more insulin. More insulin in your body causes your body to have increased insulin sensitivity. When your body has increased insulin sensitivity, you lose more fat. The brilliance of the intermittent fasting weight loss program is you skip breakfast to extend the period of your body's insulin sensitivity. This means your body is going to be on fat loss mode for a longer period. You will lose more weight.

A longer fasting mode also has a good effect on the Growth hormone levels in your body. By skipping breakfast or eating during a specific period, your body produces Growth hormone. The growth hormone is what you want your body producing when you are trying to lose weight. This is simply because the Growth hormone promotes weight loss in your body. When you are on an intermittent fasting weight loss program, your Growth hormone levels are usually at their peak. You will be losing more weight during this period. High growth hormone levels in your body also have several other health benefits. This program is simply amazing!

But What If You Didn't?

Intermittent fasting weight loss isn't necessarily a new concept. In many cultures, fasting is a regular part of life for both cultural and religious reasons. In these cases, fasting isn't done for weight loss purposes, but rather to cleanse one's body. In most cases, this method of fasting lasts anywhere from several days up to a month.

What if instead of fasting for days on end, we fast every day? Intermittent fasting weight loss methods do just that. Instead of fasting for days or weeks, the IF (Intermittent Fasting) practitioner fasts every day for anywhere from 16 - 20 hours.

A typical day eating day for most people is something like the following:

- 8:00 AM Breakfast
- Noon Lunch
- 7:00 PM Dinner

Perhaps A Light Snack Before Bed.

This schedule means that eating is spread out over a 12+ hour eating window which allows for a lot of time for overeating. Intermittent fasting allows you to eat relatively the same amounts of food, just within a compressed timeframe. An intermittent fasting weight loss schedule would look something like the following:

- 10:00 AM Breakfast
- 2:00 PM Lunch
- 6:00 PM Dinner

What we've effectively done is compress the eating window to 8 hours. Outside of the 8-hour window, nothing but water should be consumed. This has several major benefits. For starters, you'll eat less food because most people typically don't digest their food quickly enough to where they're able to consume the same amount of food that they would in a larger eating window. Eating less food while expending the same amount of effort daily will equal weight loss. Additionally, because more water is being consumed, your body has more opportunities to flush excess sodium and waste material.

Does Intermittent Fasting Work?

I've used it to consistently drop fat while preserving muscle and strength gains. There's a mental adjustment period of about 2 weeks. This is the time that it typically takes your body and mind to become used to the changes in eating. After two weeks, any hunger cravings will begin to subside.

Intermittent Fasting Bodybuilding

It is no secret that intermittent fasting helps rejuvenate the body and the fitness of a person, during intermittent fasting the person consumes only water, juices, or other low-calorie substances. It signifies a period of eating followed by a period of no eating. However, having water alone during the fasting helps to clean the body and drive out the impurities inside the body. In many cultures, especially the Chinese, intermittent fasting is more or less made compulsory to everyone, which enables people from those parts of the world to be highly agile and fit.

Intermittent Fasting Bodybuilding And The Joy Of It

Fasting and bodybuilding are often related to each other, to build the body must be fit, for the body to be fit, one of the natural ways or the most effective way is intermittent fasting, as it helps in driving away the impurities of the body and gives the various organs that participate in the digestion of food their quota of much-needed rest. Hence the person will start feeling more and more comfortable and happy with himself, this inbound feeling of wellness induces the confidence in the person and motivates him to build the body. Intermittent fasting bodybuilding hence is a natural way of improving one's fitness levels.

Points To Be Taken Care Of During Intermittent Fasting Bodybuilding

1. For beginners, the concept of intermittent fasting bodybuilding may seem to be a Herculean task, and may easily give up in no time, but it has to be understood that fasting at regular intervals of time helps oneself and boosts his confidence over some time. The perseverance has to be maintained to get the optimum results.

2. There is another tendency which we should be very wary of, and it is not to go overboard and strain yourself. Often people in a hurry to get fit and build the body of their dreams, fast too much that they fall sick, it should be avoided.

3. This can be avoided by keeping an eye out for the various hints and clues the body gives you. Like you should go and eat something and some food once you start feeling very giddy or a bit too tired or any other symbols that the body sends to indicate it's in dire need of some calories.

There is no point in fasting for a while and then shoving yourself with calories immediately after you have finished your fasting, instead slowly start taking in calories and exercise in the desired manner, making sure not to hurt yourself or overdo the exercises. Fasting & bodybuilding are one of the oldest and the time tested methods of purifying one's own body and hence maintain it in proper condition. This helps you maintain your body in shape and also gives you the much-needed confidence about yourself, above all it makes you realize the value of food and the importance of it.

Advantages Of Intermittent Fasting

Intermittent fasting is becoming more and more popular as a weight-loss and health management tool. It has several important advantages over other approaches. Here are five of them.

1. Counting calories is unnecessary on intermittent fasting. Almost all dietary approaches involve counting calories. While this may be necessary following these short-term eating plans, it is almost impossible to do this long-term. This means that when the "diet" is over, the classical rebound fat gain is just around the corner after a period of rigidly controlling all food.

2. You don't have to go hungry on intermittent fasting. When you are eating all your daily calories in a window of several hours, it becomes much more difficult to overeat when compared to a traditional grazing approach. If you are fasting, you are not worrying about whether a snack is okay or not. Fasting is not eating and when you break the fast, you eat if you are hungry. Simple!

3. Your body doesn't try to hang on to its fat stores when intermittent fasting. Most dietary approaches are necessarily restrictive. Your body is permanently deprived of enough food and reacts by going into starvation mode. It hangs on to all your fat stores and slows down your metabolism, exactly the opposite of what we want. However, when you can eat to satisfaction as is the case on a fasting diet, your body responds by continuing to drop body fat.

4. An intermittent fasting diet is less restrictive than other diets. Let's be clear here if your idea of good food is a burger and fries, nothing is going to help you until you change your perception. However, it is perfectly possible and even helpful to have some leeway in what you eat. Sure, start with your protein and veggies, but some of what you like has some interesting and positive hormonal effects if you are trying to get lean or even build some muscle.

5. An intermittent fasting diet adapts to you. This is the real beauty of this approach. Instead of trying to find exactly the right number of grams of carbs or whatever at 10 am, you fit your daily fast to your life and goals. Some find a 16 hour fast from evening until the next day at lunchtime works best. Others prefer a 24-hour cycle or even a 4-hour eating window. All of these are possible and have different advantages. It is a lifestyle rather than a diet.

Advice For Women Over 50

Intermittent fasting, because of its wide range of benefits, has turned out to be a trending practice in recent years. And, when practiced in the proper way, it can pro- vide you with some amazing results. Well, intermittent fasting can also help women who are over the age of 50, but for them, it might be a bit tough to carry on with the process just because of their age. So, for helping you in the journey, here is a list of some advice that can help you in reaching your goals of intermittent fast- ing easily and effectively.

Exercising Along With Fasting

Deciding to workout at the time of fasting can help you in various ways. It helps in increasing the fat burning rate. It has been found that if you even opt for some of the simplest exercises right before your breakfast instead of just exercising after having your breakfast, it can readily help in burning 25% of more body fat. When you exercise while keeping on with the fast, you can also develop more lean mus- cle. Having more lean muscles indicates better performance of the body. When you have more lean muscle, your body will try to burn out more calories not only at the time of exercising but throughout the entire day as your muscles will require more fuel in place of fat. Also, as you exercise while fasting, it can readily improve the insulin sensitivity of your body. Insulin is a hormone that is responsible for looking after the glucose in your blood. But, did you know that insulin indicates your body when to start with fat accumulation? Insulin is also responsible for indicating all the muscles in the body to soak up all the glucose that is available in the blood and store it as fuel for later usage. When you keep working out at the time of your fasting window, your body will tend to become more sensitive to insulin, which means it will lead to

easier weight loss, proper blood sugar levels, and also proper control over body glucose. But, remember not to start with workout just like that at the very beginning. You will need to properly listen to the responses of your body in the first place. You are also required to get accustomed to the routine of fasting before you opt for exer- cising at the time of fasting. Do not overdo as you start with it as a beginner. If you think of starting with it intensely from the very beginning, it might end up in a lower blood sugar level. Notice if you are having any kind of feelings of weakness, dizziness, brain fog, etc. If you want you can also include some electrolyte drink for the beginning phase.

Keeping The Right Mindset

No matter what you do in your life, having the right mindset is of utter importance every time when you want to achieve something. Any kind of new step that you are deciding to take or a new journey that you are thinking to start, you cannot succeed in the absence of the proper mindset. Not having the proper mindset is the primary reason why most of the people fail to continue with the process of intermittent fasting. They just give up by taking the first step as they are not focused. If you are thinking about the overall process of intermittent fasting as only a single-time pro- gram, there is a 95% chance that you will fail in it. For getting the progressive na- ture of results from the process, you need to think about it in a different way.

Set your mind in a way that makes you adopt intermittent fasting as an important process of your daily lifestyle. Be consistent with the process by making it an active part of your daily life.

Fasting After Dinner

Intermittent fasting is a very flexible process where people can decide on the type of fasting that they want to perform. You have already learned about the various types of intermittent fasting in the previous chapters. You also know the basics of all of them. Among all the various types of intermittent fasting that are available today, fasting after having your dinner is often considered as the most beneficial one. What exactly is the reason behind thinking so? The main reason behind this whole concept is obvious. As you start with the process of fasting after completing your dinner, you will have no work to do and just spend 90% of the time in your bed at night, having proper sleep. If you are following the 16/8 method of inter- mittent fasting, you can watch a movie or read a book for about three hours and then sleep for the remaining nine hours. You will be fasting for 12 hours contin- uously without having any kind of knowledge about it. That is why the 16/8 method is often regarded as the easiest method of intermittent fasting and is also easier for all beginners. With this advice, you can bring about a change in your lifestyle and make it easier and healthier. You can also improve your adherence to the daily diet. You will also be having more control over all your crav- ings and hunger.

Keeping Yourself Busy

You can actually break all the barriers with this. When you get bored or have noth- ing to do, you will tend to look out for some snacks or some food items on which you can munch on. Boredom can very easily creep in your mind and also comes with the power of easily breaking your fast, especially with some sort of food item that is not actually healthy for you and the diet. We all love watching Netflix, isn't it? It is one of the most common scenarios when you will want to have something on which you can munch on for breaking the monotony. But, what exactly results in this form of action? The answer to this very question is nothing but dopamine.

Dopamine is a hormone that can provide you with a feeling of happiness as you provide something that you want to yourself. The feeling that you have immediately after having your favorite snacks does not only take place with you. We all experience this feeling. This hormone can readily make it tough to carry on with the fast. So, what is the solution to this? You need to keep yourself and your mind busy with something that will not be having any na- ture of relation to food items. Every time when you feel like having some snacks in the middle of your fast, try shifting your focus onto something like a really inter- esting TV show or get indulged in some serious work. The main motive is to stay as busy as you can.

Going For Satiating Meals

Right after starting with the process of fasting, you need to note that if you cannot have satiating meals, you might end up feeling demotivated no matter how hard you try to stick to your overall fasting routine. This is the only way by which 90% of the people lose their motivation for carrying on the process of intermittent fasting. As you decide all your meals that you are going to have during this period in a proper way, you can have an easy time in properly maintaining your overall fasting regime. You can think of the regular diet in this pattern:

•A very simple nature of egg recipe for your breakfast time.

•Any bland type of chicken or fish dish added with various types of veggies

that will not be attracting you in any possible ways for your lunch.

•Right after getting done with your exercises, having protein supplements.

•A similar kind of bland dish for your dinner time.

In case you have enough time in your routine, you can also include various types of fruits and nuts for your snacks. This type of planning for all your meals will very obviously end up in dissatisfaction with your overall diet. You might also think of giving up the process. Additionally, this type of meal plan can also give you the worst nature of cravings. So, what can be done to it?

•You can remove breakfast from your daily meal routine. Just try to sustain on
water or coffee or any other kind of drink that has low or zero calories.
•For the lunch meal, you can carry on with a similar type of band chicken of
fish meal. But, this time try to pair it up with something that you really love, for instance, marinate your fish or chicken with BBQ seasoning.
•Take some sort of protein shake or supplement after getting done with the
workout session.
•If you want or if you are really willing to, you can go out for dinner. But
remember that you cannot have any type of processed foods

Benefits of Intermittent

Helps Reduce Weight

There are a lot of diet plans out there and most of them talk about reducing your calorific intake and replace meals. The problem is that when the diet is over and you have reached your goal it is easy to go back to old habits and put the weight back on. Intermittent fasting is more of a lifestyle change and a slow burn diet. One of the most popular intermittent fasting diets is the 5:2 plan. Here you eat normally for 5 days and reduce your calorie intake for the other 2. There are many ways you can do this, you can eat nothing for 24 hours or reduce calorie intake to just drink fluids or very light meals. Your 2 days shouldn't be back to back, spread them throughout the week.

Blood Pressure, Insulin, and Cholesterol

Numerous studies have shown that intermittent fasting will help reduce Cholesterol and Insulin which helps break down body fat and boost your energy. Furthermore, intermittent fasting can reduce the body's resistance to insulin which significantly lowers the risk of type 2 diabetes. Intermittent fasting has shown to relieve stress and high blood pressure, which are both key risks for heart disease. When we fast a few days a week the body goes through a process that renews old cells and provides protection against various diseases.

Effect On The Brain

Intermittent fasting can help the brain recover quickly and stay healthy. Reduction in blood sugar and reduced inflammation increase your brain hormones which will keep you alert and focused. As well as helping the brain prevents diseases that affect the brain such as Alzheimer's. Fasting can help delay the onset of this degenerative disease.

Potential Risks Of Fasting

The most common risk of intermittent fasting is dehydration. If you are consuming less than your body is taking on less water, it is very important you don't forget to drink on the days you do not eat. Water is essential and black coffee is often used if you get bored with plain water. With no food going in the stomach you are at risk from heartburn from stomach acid and long-term ulcers that can occur if stomach acid builds up against the stomach walls.

The mental side of fasting also has to be considered. If you fast 2 days a week don't overindulge on the other 5, keep to normal meals or it could lead someone to psychological disorders such as bulimia. You also need to be sure you are eating the right nutrients and minerals. Continue to eat fruit and vegetables. If you don't eat for 2 days, make sure the other 5 you are eating enough fruit and vegetables and not just binge or convenience foods.

Tips For Maintaining Intermittent Fasting

It can be challenging to stick to an intermittent fasting program. The following tips may help people stay on track and maximize the benefits of intermittent fasting:

i. Staying Hydrated

Drink lots of water and calorie-free drinks, such as herbal teas, throughout the day.

ii. Avoiding Obsessing Over Food.

Plan plenty of distractions on fasting days to avoid thinking about food, such as catching up on paperwork or going to see a movie.

iii. Resting And Relaxing.

Avoid strenuous activities on fasting days, although light exercise such as yoga may be beneficial.

iv. Making Every Calorie Count.

If the chosen plan allows some calories during fasting periods, select nutrient-dense foods that are rich in protein, fiber, and healthful fats. Examples include beans, lentils, eggs, fish, nuts, and avocado.

v. Eating High-Volume Foods

Select filling yet low-calorie foods, which include popcorn, raw vegetables, and fruits with high water content, such as grapes and melon.

vi. Increasing The Taste Without The Calories.

Season meals generously with garlic, herbs, spices, or vinegar. These foods are extremely low in calories yet are full of flavor, which may help to reduce feelings of hunger.

vii. Choosing Nutrient-Dense Foods After The Fasting Period.

Eating foods that are high in fiber, vitamins, minerals, and other nutrients helps to keep blood sugar levels steady and prevent nutrient deficiencies. A balanced diet will also contribute to weight loss and overall health. Think about what you genuinely want from Intermittent fasting. Focus on the quality of the process, not the outcome.

viii. Break Your Fast With A Normal Sized Meal

We touched on this earlier when we talked about how IF isn't an excuse to eat whatever you want. As with every other diet out there, IF only works for fat loss or muscle building if you maintain the appropriate calorie deficit or surplus. This means when it comes time to break your fast you don't want to throw caution the wind, particularly when your goal is fat loss.

Yes, skipping breakfast frees up calories to give you more freedom for your other meals but if you go too crazy then you'll undo the calorie deficit you worked so hard to create. Now, your meal size when breaking your fast will depend on whether you've just worked out or are working out later in the day.

ix. Stick To A Routine

Having a routine makes it easier to stick to your IF schedule because when you discover what works for you and stick to it every day you remove the doubt and second-guessing from the equation. All you have to do is follow-through. Not mention that establishing a routine helps to remove decision fatigue. Which is the term given to the deterioration of your ability to make decisions after a prolonged period of making decisions. What this means is that if you're continually having to make decisions like:

- What you'll eat
- When you'll eat it
- When you have time to cook it
- If it fits your calories and macros

x. Start Your Fast After Dinner

Where you're doing daily or weekly fasts, one of the best tips I can give you is to start your fast after dinner. Doing this means you'll spend a big chunk of your fasting period asleep. Particularly when using a daily fasting setup like 16:8 if you start fasting after dinner and then:

- Spend 1 – 3 hours watching TV or other evening activities
- Spend 6 – 9 hours asleep

You've already fasted for anywhere from 7 to 12 hours, making a 16-hour much more manageable. This means:

- Increased dietary adherence
- Easier lifestyle
- More manageable hunger

xi. Don't keep Foods In The House That You Might Binge on.

This is a cardinal rule for any healthy eating plan, and intermittent fasting is no different. Fasting results in smaller appetites for many people, but that doesn't mean you can't override your hunger cues to seriously overeat a favorite snack and even give yourself "permission" to do so because you fasted all day.

Intermittent Fasting Is A Great Way To:

- Go deeper into the psychological and physical experience of true hunger;
- Learn the difference between "head hunger" and "body hunger;"
- Learn not to fear hunger;
- Improve insulin sensitivity and re-calibrate your body's use of stored fuel;
- Respect the process and privilege of eating;
- Learn more about your own body;
- Lose fat, if you are careful about it; and,

- Take a break from the work of food prep and the obligation to eat.

Intermittent Fasting Is Not Healthy If:

- You're using the pretext of "health" as a way to have an eating disorder or rigidly control your food intake (which is the same thing);
- You fast too often, too long;
- You're also overexercising or not getting enough sleep (i.e., under too much additional physiological stress);
- You're using a lot of supplements, legal or otherwise, to kill your appetite so you can make it through your fasts;
- You're food-obsessed and binge during your non-fasting periods; and,
- You use IF as a way to "compensate" for poor food choices or over-eating.

CHAPTER 2: INTERMITTENT FASTING TYPES

When it comes to intermittent fasting, there is no single method that fits everyone. The most important thing is finding a program that fits your lifestyle, health, and goals a program you can actually stick to in the long run. In this book, we will introduce you to some of the most popular forms of fasting in detail.

The Warrior Diet

The 20:4 intermittent fasting method, also known as the Warrior Diet.The Warrior Diet is a relatively extreme form of intermittent fasting. It is where you fast for 20 hours and have your meals within the remaining 4 hours. During the fast, you are not allowed to consume any snacks or beverages that have calories. Sleep usually counts as part of the fast. This diet, unlike other programs that do not allow the intake of carbohydrates, often stresses the idea of timing what you consume and when to drink or eat.

When you fast for long hours like, for example, in the Warrior Diet, which is 20 hours, insulin will automatically stay low for a more extended period. All you can have during this time is coffee, tea, or any other beverage that does not have calories. It is not a must for you to limit the eating window to evenings only like it was done before; you can tailor-make your fasting and eating window according to your preferences.

The Warrior Diet involves eating very little, usually just a few servings of raw fruit and vegetables, during a 20-hour fasting window, then eating one large meal at night. The eating window is usually only around 4 hours. This form of fasting may be best for people who have tried other forms of intermittent fasting already. It allows you to eat small portions of certain food types at dinner. During that dinner period, you should also work out. At the end of the day, you would have a feeding window.

During the 4-hour eating phase, people should make sure they consume plenty of vegetables, proteins, and healthful fats. They should also include some carbohydrates. Although it is possible to eat some foods during the fasting period, it can be challenging to stick to the strict guidelines on when and what to eat in the long term. Also, some people struggle with eating such a large meal so close to bedtime.

There is also a risk that people on this diet will not eat enough nutrients, such as fiber. This can increase the risk of cancer and have an adverse effect on digestive and immune health. When you do the 20:4 fasting techniques, you are sure to be more focused and have more energy. The first days of the fast, you may experience hunger pangs, but when you go on with the fasting, the hunger will tremendously reduce. This technique of intermittent fasting can quickly become addictive once you see the mental clarity that comes with it.

Above all intermittent fasting techniques, the worrier's diet seems to be the strictest because it only has a 4-hour eating window, and most people are unable to adhere to that. As we said earlier, you can tailor-make the fast to suit you. Some people who are fasting, prefer to drink morning coffee and leave the 4 hour eating period for evenings. However, some find themselves hungrier during the day hence scheduling their eating window at lunch hour.

What you are advised is that it does not matter what time you choose your eating period to be. What matters is that you stick to an extremely low carb diet. Low carbohydrates usually make the hunger pangs to go down, and this will help you get through the 20 hours of fasting. For the

20 hour fast, it is usually advised to stick to the ketogenic diet by eating meals such as:

- For the starches: Sweet potatoes, corn, and potatoes.
- For proteins: Lean meat, fish, chicken, and eggs are allowed.
- Oats, bread, pasta
- For oils, you can use olive oil
- Milk, cheese, and yogurt.
- Cauliflower, zucchini, leafy veggies.

THE WARRIOR DIET

	DAY 1	DAY 2	DAY 3	DAY 4	DAY 5	DAY 6	DAY 7
Midnight 4 AM 8 AM 12 PM	Eating only small amounts of vegetables and fruits	Eating only small amounts of vegetables and fruits	Eating only small amounts of vegetables and fruits	Eating only small amounts of vegetables and fruits	Eating only small amounts of vegetables and fruits	Eating only small amounts of vegetables and fruits	Eating only small amounts of vegetables and fruits
4 PM	Large meal	Large meal	Large meal	Large meal	Large meal	Large meal	Large meal
8 PM Midnight							

Always choose foods higher in protein to consume fewer fats. Some people have a heavy meal at the beginning of the eating window, and when the eating window is almost over, they have a simple snack. Ensure that you have your meals early enough so when you have your heavy meal, you don't get so full that you feel uncomfortable when going to bed.

Glycogen, a carbohydrate in storage form, will be used up when the body has not had anything and especially during your feeding period when you only had ketogenic foods. Throughout the fasting period, the body will begin to burn more body fat when the glycogen finishes. The longer you stay without eating, the better because your insulin levels will remain low, and this will ensure that the liver uses your body fat to fuel itself.

When your blood glucose is low, the liver will be signaled by the little insulin prompting it to dump its glycogen into the bloodstream. The 20:4 fasting techniques have many side effects and benefits. One of the advantages is you will have reduced cholesterol and inflammation. We have seen all the benefits of inflammation on the other chapters above. When on the 20:4 diet, you will improve mental clarity, and your concentration will be top-notch.

Your blood glucose levels will also increase tremendously. If you were used to eating lots of carbohydrates, you will see significant changes such as you will not be feeling hungry and craving unhealthy meals. Cases of insulin resistance can be corrected using the 20:4 fasting technique. Fat stores are made more accessible to the liver by reducing your food intake, hence lowering your insulin levels.

The 5:2 fast

This is one of the most popular methods of fasting. The 5:2 diet gets its name because is it involves eating regularly for 5 days of the week while drastically limiting caloric intake on the other 2 two days. While the 5:2 diet is a popular form of intermittent fasting, the term fasting is slightly misleading. Unlike a true fast, which involves eating nothing for a set amount of time, the goal of the 5:2 diet is to cut caloric intake on fasting days to 25 percent or just one-quarter of a person's regular intake on the remaining days. For example, a person who regularly eats about 2,000 calories per day would eat 500 calories on fasting days.

Importantly, fasting days are not consecutive because it is vital to give the body the calories and nutrients it needs to thrive. People typically space their fasting days out, for example, by taking their reduced-calorie days on Monday and Thursday or Wednesday and Saturday. Part of the diet's appeal is this flexibility. Instead of severely restricting the foods a person can eat, the 5:2 diet focuses on strict caloric restriction on only 2 days of the week. This may help some people feel more satisfied with their diet, as they will not feel they are missing out all the time.

The 5 normal days of the 5:2 diet should still involve a healthful diet, however. Loading up on sugary or processed foods for 5 days

THE 5:2 DIET

DAY 1	DAY 2	DAY 3	DAY 4	DAY 5	DAY 6	DAY 7
Eats normally	Women: 500 calories Men: 600 calories	Eats normally	Eats normally	Women: 500 calories Men: 600 calories	Eats normally	Eats normally

and then having a small break may not be as helpful as keeping a trend of clean eating during the entire week.

This fasting method is highly flexible; you can choose whichever two days you prefer. However, we highly recommend including at least one non-fasting day in between those two days. The 500-600 calories can be either consumed in a single meal or spread out into multiple meals over the course of the day.

Women who eat two meals a day should break it down to 250 calories per meal, and men should raise this number to 300 calories. This one is quite easy to follow, especially if you know you have two days per week where you tend to be less physically active, meaning you also have to consume fewer calories for energy.

12-Hour Fasts

This one is probably the most beginner-friendly fasting method. A 12-hour fast means that you eat within the first 12 hours of the day and abstain from food for the next 12 hours. For example, if you eat three meals a day from 8 a.m. to 8 p.m., then you should fast from 8 p.m. to 8 a.m. This method is easy to follow and provides amazing results in the long run. Though it is said that your body is out of blood sugar 8 hours after your last meal. That means if you follow a 12-hour fasting method, you will be burning fat for 4 hours only. Of course, that's better than nothing but keep in mind, that you can start with this one, see how you're doing and then extend your fasting time bit by bit until you're ready to follow 16:8 method!

The 12-Hour Fasting Techniques Have Many Health Benefits.

Detoxification

The body is known to use lots of energy to ensure it removes toxins from your body. The body usually focuses on eliminating toxins and healing itself when it is not digesting food, and that's why the 12 hour fast is essential. Detoxification is optimized because when you go on the loose, the body will focus on repairing itself.

Helps In Managing Weight

For the body to burn its glycogen supply, it will take roughly 8 hours. When the number of glycogen finishes, the body will use the stored fats to produce energy. It becomes a bit hard for the body to burn fat when someone eats throughout the whole day. When you stay for 12 hours without eating, the body taps into the fat reserve forcefully to produce energy.

Research Shows That Fasting Can Significantly Improve The Health Of The Mitochondria

Brain health immensely enhances through the support of mitochondrial health. Recent studies have also demonstrated that progressive brain disorders might be prevented thanks to intermittent fasting.

16:8 intermittent fasting

16:8 intermittent fasting, which people sometimes call the 16:8 diet or 16:8 plan, is a popular type of fasting. People who follow this eating plan will fast for 16 hours a day and consume all of their calories during the remaining 8 hours. Suggested benefits of the 16:8 plan include weight loss and fat loss, as well as the prevention of type 2 diabetes and other obesity-associated conditions. 16:8 intermittent fasting is a form of time-restricted fasting. It involves consuming foods during an 8-hour window and avoiding food, or fasting, for the remaining 16 hours each day.

16-hour fasts are a bit more complex than 12-hour fasts, but in return, they lead to even better results. As the title implies, you should hold off from any food for 16 hours and eat during the remaining 8 hours of the day. When following this method of fasting, you have to consume lots of high-protein foods and eat carbohydrates on rotation. If you exercise, you should try to be strategic with your nutrient intake. This means that the majority of your carbohydrates should be consumed immediately after a workout. For example, if you eat from 11 a.m. to 7 p.m., then during that period you should eat two to four or five meals and fast from 7 p.m. to 11 a.m.

When following this method of fasting, some people choose to skip the morning meal every day and have snacks before other meals instead. This fasting method would probably be the most popular one and it has the best easy-to-follow and effectiveness ratio! Some people believe that this method works by supporting the body's circadian rhythm, which is its internal clock.

Most people who follow the 16:8 plan abstain from food at night and for part of the morning and evening. They tend to consume their daily calories during the middle of the day. There are no restrictions on the types or amounts of food a person can eat during the 8-hour window. This flexibility makes the plan relatively easy to follow.

THE 16/8 METHOD

	DAY 1	DAY 2	DAY 3	DAY 4	DAY 5	DAY 6	DAY 7
Midnight 4 AM 8 AM	FAST	FAST	FAST	FAST	FAST	FAST	FAST
12 PM	First meal	First meal	First meal	First meal	First meal	First meal	First meal
4 PM	Last meal by 8pm	Last meal by 8pm	Last meal by 8pm	Last meal by 8pm	Last meal by 8pm	Last meal by 8pm	Last meal by 8pm
8 PM Midnight	FAST	FAST	FAST	FAST	FAST	FAST	FAST

How To Do It

The easiest way to follow the 16:8 diet is to choose a 16-hour fasting window that includes the time that a person spends sleeping. Some experts advise finishing food consumption in the early evening, as metabolism slows down after this time. However, this is not feasible for everyone. Some people may not be able to consume their evening meal until 7 p.m. or later. Even so, it is best to avoid food for 2–3 hours before bed. People may choose one of the following 8-hour eating windows:

- 9 a.m. to 5 p.m.
- 10 a.m. to 6 p.m.
- noon to 8 p.m.

Within this timeframe, people can eat their meals and snacks at convenient times. Eating regularly is important to prevent blood sugar peaks and dips and to avoid excessive hunger. Some people may need to experiment to find the best eating window and mealtimes for their lifestyle.

Recommended Foods And Tips

While the 16:8 intermittent fasting plan does not specify which foods to eat and avoid, it is beneficial to focus on healthful eating and to limit or avoid junk foods. The consumption of too much unhealthful food may cause weight gain and contribute to disease.

A Balanced Diet Focuses Primarily On:

- Fruits and vegetables, which can be fresh, frozen, or canned (in water)
- Whole grains, including quinoa, brown rice, oats, and barley
- Lean protein sources, such as poultry, fish, beans, lentils, tofu, nuts, seeds, low fat cottage cheese, and eggs
- Healthful fats from fatty fish, olives, olive oil, coconuts, avocados, nuts, and seeds
- Fruits, vegetables, and whole grains are high in fiber, so they can help keep a person feeling full and satisfied. Healthful fats and proteins can also contribute to satiety.

Beverages can play a role in satiety for those following the 16:8 intermittent fasting diet. Drinking water regularly throughout the day can help reduce calorie intake because people often mistake thirst for hunger. The 16:8 diet plan permits the consumption of calorie-free drinks such as water and unsweetened tea and coffee during the 16-hour fasting window. It is important to consume fluids regularly to avoid dehydration.

Tips

People may find it easier to stick to the 16:8 diet when they follow these tips:

- Drinking cinnamon herbal tea during the fasting period, as it may suppress the appetite
- Consuming water regularly throughout the day
- Watching less television to reduce exposure to images of food, which may stimulate a sense of hunger
- Exercising just before or during the eating window, as exercise can trigger hunger
- Practicing mindful eating when consuming meals
- Trying meditation during the fasting period to allow hunger pangs to pass

Weekly Intermittent Fasting

One of the best ways to get started with intermittent fasting is to do it once per week or once per month. The occasional fast has been shown to lead to many of the benefits of fasting we've already talked about, so even if you don't use it to cut down on calories consistently there are still many other health benefits of fasting.

In this example, lunch on Monday is your last meal of the day. You then fast until lunch on Tuesday. This schedule has the advantage of allowing you to eat everyday of the week while still reaping the benefits of fasting for 24 hours. It's also less likely that you'll lose weight because you are only cutting out two meals per week. So, if you're looking to bulk up or keep weight on, then this is a great option.

Meal Skipping

This flexible approach to intermittent fasting may be good for beginners. It involves occasionally skipping meals. People can decide which meals to skip according to their level of hunger or time restraints. However, it is important to eat healthful foods at each meal. Meal skipping is likely to be most successful when individuals monitor and respond to their body's hunger signals. Essentially, people using this style of intermittent fasting will eat when they are hungry and skip meals when they are not. This may feel more natural for some people than the other fasting methods.

Eat-Stop-Eat: Do A 24-Hour Fast, Once Or Twice A Week

Eat-Stop-Eat involves a 24-hour fast, either once or twice per week. This method was popularized by fitness expert Brad Pilon and has been quite popular for a few years. By fasting from dinner one day to dinner the next day, this amounts to a full 24-hour fast. For example, if you finish dinner at 7 p.m. Monday and don't eat

until dinner at 7 p.m. the next day, you've just done a full 24-hour fast.

EAT-STOP-EAT

DAY 1	DAY 2	DAY 3	DAY 4	DAY 5	DAY 6	DAY 7
Eats normally	24-hour fast	Eats normally	Eats normally	24-hour fast	Eats normally	Eats normally

You can also fast from breakfast to breakfast or lunch to lunch. The end result is the same. Water, coffee, and other noncaloric beverages are allowed during the fast, but no solid foods are permitted. If you're doing this to lose weight, it's very important that you eat normally during the eating periods. As in, eat the same amount of food as if you had do been fasting at all. The potential downside of this method is that a full 24-hour fast may be fairly difficult for many people. However, you don't need to go all-in right away. Starting with 14-16 hours and then moving upward from there is fine.

The 23:1 Fasting Technique

This technique is also known as OMAD, which stands for one meal per day. People can lose weight by having one meal per day, which is intermittent fasting. It means that you will fast for 23 hours then have a 1 hour period where you can have your lunch. During the fast, you are only allowed to take beverages with zero calories such as coffee, black tea, or green tea, whereas, during your eating period, you can have your regular meals.

It is, however, advisable to feed on meals that are rich in nutrients.

SPONTANEOUS MEAL SKIPPING

	DAY 1	DAY 2	DAY 3	DAY 4	DAY 5	DAY 6	DAY 7
Breakfast	Breakfast	Skipped Meal	Breakfast	Breakfast	Breakfast	Breakfast	Breakfast
Lunch	Lunch	Lunch	Lunch	Lunch	Lunch	Lunch	Lunch
Dinner	Dinner	Dinner	Dinner	Dinner	Skipped Meal	Dinner	Dinner

Apart from weight loss, the 23:1 fasting technique has a lot of health benefits. Some of the health benefits are:

- Decreased rates of contracting diseases
- The human growth hormone increases
- The inflammations levels are lowered drastically
- Autophagy
- Has a positive impact on sleeping patterns of people who are obese

- It helps people with diabetes type 2 to lower their blood sugar levels.

This diet is not as hard to follow because the number of calories is not counted. The effects of the 23; 1 cycle may be a bit different in men because of unlike women, they do not go through hormonal cycles. Enhancement of ketosis is also one of the benefits of the 23: 1-hour fasting technique. OMAD is usually a prolonged fast, and thus, it often maximizes n benefits such as anti-inflammatory, fat-burning, and autophagy. Due to the long hours without food, the 23:1 fasting technique might have some downside.

Some of the disadvantages are:

Not Getting Enough Food.

The OMAD diet or 23:1 diet means you fast for long hours, which makes it hard at times for the body to get enough food. For you to ensure you are well sorted during the fasting window, always ensure you eat food that has calories. Ensure the calories you eat are enough for your weight, age, and the type of activities you carry out daily. Also, ensure that the meal you eat during your feeding period is one heavy meal. When you are not used to intermittent fasting, the 23:1, not getting enough food may cause you to lose focus.

Another Downside Of OMAD Is That It Can Cause Extreme Hunger.

Due to the long periods without food, a person may get so hungry when fasting and this might lead to temptations of feeding on unhealthy foods when you are only supposed to feed on foods that don't have calories.

Feeling Weak.

Due to the more extended fasting periods and having just a meal in a day may cause a person to feel weak. It is because the food intake will have decreased, and hence making the body to produce energy that is not enough eventually will lead to fatigue.

Getting Fewer Nutrients

Studies have proved that on a day to day basis, a female adult needs 2500 calories, whereas a man needs 2000 calories. When you are on the OMAD or the 23; 1 technique of fasting, you only get only 750 calories, hence making a person hungry. To get nutrients such as calcium that usually are not found in the meals, a person is advised to eat yogurt or drink milk.

It Causes A Person To Be Irritable

A person may become easily irritated because of hunger. It is also easy for the person to not concentrate and even have mood swings. For those who are just starting the intermittent fasting, the OMAD or 23:1 fasting technique is not advisable. You can begin by doing the most straightforward routines, like lowering your sugar intake. Also, try and put your focus on healthy fats and take lots of veggies and clean proteins which will act as a stepping stone towards OMAD fasting.

Alternate Day Intermittent Fasting

Whether you are looking for a powerful way to shed some pounds or simply improve your general health, alternate day fasting is just what you need. A growing body of evidence suggests that alternate-day fasting not only helps with weight loss but also promotes heart health in both normal weight and overweight individuals. That said, it also comes with some risks you should not ignore.

Alternate day fasting is a time-restricted eating method in which you fast one day and eat normally the next day. Simply put, you have alternating "fasting days" and "feeding days." On the fasting days, you may consume no calories or about 500 calories, which contributes to approximately one-fourth of your daily calorie needs. On the feeding days, you can stick to your normal eating habits and consume the foods/drinks you want.

Thus, it is critically important to learn the benefits and drawbacks of this method of fasting, especially if you have just started to fast. Doing so will help maximize the results and cut down the chances of potential complications. Alternate day intermittent fasting incorporates longer fasting periods on alternating days throughout the week.

Alternate Day Fasting Benefits

Mounting scientific evidence supports the role of alternate day fasting in weight reduction, decreased risk of heart disease, and improved blood glucose and fat levels. Interestingly, one case report even goes as far as to say that planned intermittent fasting including ADF may help reverse type II diabetes. While it might be too early to jump to a conclusion regarding diabetes reversal, scientists are sure of ADF's incredible health benefits.

These include:

Improved Heart Health

Heart disease is the leading cause of death globally. Estimates suggest that diseases of the heart and blood vessels accounted for more than one-third of deaths globally in 2018. Alternate day fasting helps reduce the risk of heart disease in many ways. It:

- Promotes weight loss;
- Decreases the blood levels of the bad cholesterol (LDL);
- Increases the blood levels of the good cholesterol (HDL);
- Decreases blood pressure;
- Significantly decreases the blood levels of "harmful" fats (triglycerides).

Better Blood Sugar Control

High blood sugar levels occur when the body fails to produce enough insulin, or cannot properly use available insulin (insulin resistance). In any case, persistently high sugar levels can lead to diabetes. Studies have shown short-term alternate day fasting or other forms of intermittent fasting can help reduce fasting blood glucose levels. ADF works by reducing the blood levels of insulin and increasing insulin sensitivity.

Alternate Day Fasting Promotes Autophagy

Both long-term and short-term fasting is known to trigger autophagy in the body. Autophagy is a destructive process that recycles unused, damaged, and potentially harmful cell components. In simple terms, autophagy is the body's way of clearing unwanted substances from the cells. Autophagy is thought to reduce the risk of many diseases. These include infections, heart disease, obesity, and cancer.

For example, in the graphic below you would eat dinner on Monday night and then not eat again until Tuesday evening. On Wednesday, however, you would eat all day and then start the 24–hour fasting cycle again after dinner on Wednesday evening. This allows you to get long fast periods on a consistent basis while also eating at least one meal every day of the week.

ALTERNATE-DAY FASTING

DAY 1	DAY 2	DAY 3	DAY 4	DAY 5	DAY 6	DAY 7
Eats normally	24-hour fast OR Eat only a few hundred calories	Eats normally	24-hour fast OR Eat only a few hundred calories	Eats normally	24-hour fast OR Eat only a few hundred calories	Eats normally

CHAPTER 3 : INTRODUCING THE 16:8 INTERMITTENT FASTING

What Is 16:8 Intermittent Fasting?

16:8 intermittent fasting is a form of time-restricted fasting. It involves consuming foods during an 8-hour window and avoiding food, or fasting, for the remaining 16 hours each day.

What Is The 16:8 Diet?

The 16:8 diet is a type of time-restricted fasting done to achieve better health or lose weight. (The 5:2 diet followed by Jimmy Kimmel, where you eat whatever you want five days a week and only consume 500 calories or less on the other two days, is also a modified form of fasting.)

On the 16:8 diet, you spend 16 hours of each day consuming nothing but unsweetened beverages like water, coffee, and tea. The remaining eight-hour window is when you eat all of your meals and snacks. Most people do this by starting a fast at night, skipping breakfast, and eating their first meal in the middle of the day. No foods are inherently off-limits during that time, but some people will follow the keto diet at mealtimes to supercharge their weight loss.

How To Do It

The easiest way to follow the 16:8 diet is to choose a 16-hour fasting window that includes the time that a person spends sleeping. Some experts advise finishing food consumption in the early evening, as metabolism slows down after this time. However, this is not feasible for everyone.

Some people may not be able to consume their evening meal until 7 p.m. or later. Even so, it is best to avoid food for 2–3 hours before bed. People may choose one of the following 8-hour eating windows:

- 9 a.m. to 5 p.m.
- 10 a.m. to 6 p.m.
- Afternoon to 8 p.m.

Within this timeframe, people can eat their meals and snacks at convenient times. Eating regularly is important to prevent blood sugar peaks and dips and to avoid excessive hunger. Some people may need to experiment to find the best eating window and mealtimes for their lifestyle.

Recommended Foods And Tips

While the 16:8 intermittent fasting plan does not specify which foods to eat and avoid, it is beneficial to focus on healthy eating and to limit or avoid junk foods. The consumption of too much unhealthful food may cause weight gain and contribute to disease.

A Balanced Diet Focuses Primarily On:

- Fruits and vegetables, which can be fresh, frozen, or canned (in water)
- Whole grains, including quinoa, brown rice, oats, and barley
- Lean protein sources, such as poultry, fish, beans, lentils, tofu, nuts, seeds, low-fat cottage cheese, and eggs
- Healthful fats from fatty fish, olives, olive oil, coconuts, avocados, nuts, and seeds
- Fruits, vegetables, and whole grains are high in fiber, so they can help keep a person feeling full and satisfied. Healthful fats and proteins can also contribute to satiety.
- Beverages can play a role in satiety for those following the 16:8 intermittent fasting diet. Drinking water

regularly throughout the day can help reduce calorie intake because people often mistake thirst for hunger.

The 16:8 diet plan permits the consumption of calorie-free drinks such as water and unsweetened tea and coffee during the 16-hour fasting window. It is important to consume fluids regularly to avoid dehydration.

Tips

People may find it easier to stick to the 16:8 diet when they follow these tips:

- Drinking cinnamon herbal tea during the fasting period, as it may suppress the appetite
- Consuming water regularly throughout the day
- Watching less television to reduce exposure to images of food, which may stimulate a sense of hunger
- Exercising just before or during the eating window, as exercise can trigger hunger
- Practicing mindful eating when consuming meals
- Trying meditation during the fasting period to allow hunger pangs to pass
- Health benefits

Study findings are sometimes contradictory and inconclusive. However, the research on intermittent fasting, including 16:8 fasting, indicates it may provide the following benefits:

Weight Loss And Fat Loss

Eating during a set period can help people reduce the number of calories that they consume. It may also help boost metabolism.

Should You Try 16:8 Fasting?

Ultimately, it's a personal choice. But there are a few beneficial behaviors you can try without committing to the riskier elements of 16-

hour fasts. The first is to better understand mindfulness and how it relates to your food choices. To get started, consider these questions when you're deciding when and what to eat:

Where Are You Physically When You Decide To Eat?

Many of us eat based on the scenario, not our hunger levels. Case in point: Raise your hand if you've ever gone to the movies after dinner and suddenly wanted popcorn? Yep, me too! By considering the moments when you eat, you may become aware of patterns you didn't notice before. Say you're a person who loves to graze during The Bachelor. If you're fasting after 8 p.m., you've automatically cut hours and subsequently, calories from your post-dinner snacking.

Are You Getting Enough Sleep?

If you've cut out late-night snacking, that alone could help you go to bed earlier a very crucial component to any weight loss plan. Getting seven hours of sleep per night has been linked to better weight management, reduced risk of chronic disease, and improved metabolism.

Are Fasting 16 Hours A Day Healthy?

Forms of intermittent fasting like the 16:8 diet rely on the concept that fasting reduces oxidative stress on the body, which can decrease inflammation and the risk of chronic diseases. It's also theorized that fasting gives your vital organs, digestive and absorptive hormones, and metabolic functions a "break," according to a recent study published in Cell Metabolism. Since our bodies secrete insulin to help our cells absorb sugar, fasting is linked to reducing our susceptibility to insulin resistance over time. (High insulin levels ultimately put us at risk for a whole host of diseases.)

I also have a much deeper concern about the disordered eating behaviors that may arise from intermittent fasting. Research shows that fasting for a period followed by a limited window for eating primes you to overeat. It's a cycle that can be difficult to get out of because it impairs our body's natural hunger cues and metabolism. Restricted eating may also lead to an increased risk of depression and anxiety.

Disease Prevention

Supporters of intermittent fasting suggest that it can prevent several conditions and diseases, including:

- Type 2 diabetes
- Heart conditions
- Some cancers
- Neurodegenerative diseases

Side Effects And Risks

16:8 intermittent fasting has some associated risks and side effects. As a result, the plan is not right for everyone.

Potential Side Effects And Risks Include:

- Hunger, weakness, and tiredness in the beginning stages of the plan
- Overeating or eating unhealthful foods during the 8-hour eating window due to excessive hunger
- Heartburn or reflux as a result of overeating

Intermittent fasting may be less beneficial for women than men. Some research on animals suggests that intermittent fasting could negatively affect female fertility. Individuals with a history of disordered eating may wish to avoid intermittent fasting. The National Eating Disorders Association warn that fasting is a risk factor for eating disorders.

The 16:8 plan may also not be suitable for those with a history of depression and anxiety. Some research indicates that short-term calorie restriction might relieve depression, but that chronic calorie restriction can have the opposite effect. More research is necessary to understand the implications of these findings.

16:8 intermittent fasting is unsuitable for those who are pregnant, breastfeeding, or trying to conceive. The National Institute on Aging concludes there is insufficient evidence to recommend any fasting diet, especially for older adults.

People who wish to try the 16:8 method or other types of intermittent fasting should talk to their doctor first, especially if they are taking medications or have:

- An underlying health condition, such as diabetes or low blood pressure
- A history of disordered eating
- A history of mental health disorders
- Anyone who has any concerns or experiences any adverse effects of the diet should see a doctor.

Diabetes

While evidence indicates the 16:8 method may be helpful for diabetes prevention, it may not be suitable for those who already have the condition. The 16:8 intermittent fasting diet is not suitable for people with type 1 diabetes. However, some people with prediabetes or type 2 diabetes may be able to try the diet under a doctor's supervision. People with diabetes who wish to try the 16:8 intermittent fasting plan should see their doctor before making changes to their eating habits.

Does It Work?

Yes but fasting offers weight loss similar to any reduction in calories. The best diet is the one where you are healthy, hydrated and living your best life. If fasting works for you, go for it.

How Do I Try Intermittent Fasting?

There are four popular fasting approaches periodic fasting, time-restricted feeding, alternate-day fasting, and the 5:2 diet. Time-restricted feeding, sometimes called daily intermittent fasting, is perhaps the easiest and most popular fasting method. Daily intermittent fasters restrict eating to certain periods each day, say 11 in the morning to 7 at night.

The fasting period is usually around 12 or more hours that, helpfully, includes time spent sleeping overnight. Periodic fasting will feel most familiar: no food or drinks with calories for 24-hour periods. Another type of fast, alternate-day fasting requires severe calorie reduction every other day. Lastly, "The 5:2 Diet" and requires fasting on two nonconsecutive days a week.

CHAPTER 4: PRECAUTIONS DURING INTERMITTENT FASTING

Healthy Foods To Eat

This means eating whole foods and avoiding the usual suspects such as sugar, processed foods, empty carbs, etc. The type of diet you choose is up to you; as long it is balanced and fits your lifestyle. For many, the Keto Diet has proven to be a great supplement to Intermittent Fasting, as it may help you burn more fat. When doing intermittent fasting, there are restrictions as to the types of foods you should eat when on your feeding window. For the intermittent fasting to be more productive, eat unprocessed foods that are high in fiber. The menus below are some of the healthy foods you should eat during intermittent fasting.

i. Avocado

Unlike other fruits high in carbohydrates, avocados contain healthy fats. Just like olive oil, avocados contain monounsaturated fats that always leave a person full for more extended periods after consumption. As much as the avocado fruit s a high percentage of fat, it also contains lots of water and fiber. The good thing about avocados is you can add them to salads. Apart from that, they also contain nutrients that are important to the body and potassium.

ii. Fish

Fish that have a few fats like salmon are significant during intermittent fasting. It is because, when you eat it, you will remain full for longer hours. Apart from quality protein and healthy fats, salmon also contains reasonable amounts of vitamin D. Iodine may also be found in fish. The nutrients found in fish are essential because they ensure the thyroid functions properly. When the thyroid functions correctly, it keeps your metabolism running at optimum. When you consume fish, you get the omega3 fatty acids that studies have shown help to reduce inflammations.

iii. Eggs

In some people, the levels of bad cholesterol increase by consuming eggs. When you are on a weight-loss mission, they are one of the best foods you can eat. It is because it has proteins and you can cook it up in minutes, and it will make you feel full for longer hours. For muscle build-up, you need as much protein as possible. You can now get all the nutrients you need on a calorie-restricted diet as eggs are always nutrient dense. Eggs also promote weight loss by suppressing the appetite during the day.

iv. Leafy Greens

Kales, collards, and spinach are some of the leafy greens that you should consume during intermittent fasting. They are usually very loaded with fiber and low in carbohydrates, making them extremely good for weight loss. You can comfortably eat a lot of leafy greens without the fear of consuming a lot of calories. The leafy greens also contain minerals and antioxidants. They are also very nutritious and have lots of vitamins. When you eat the leafy greens, you will always feel full for longer hours due to the high fiber content.

v. Whole Grains

Some whole grains are very healthy, and this is because they have loads of fiber. It will help in making you feel full for longer hours at a time. Some of the examples of whole grains are oats. Oats usually have fiber that is soluble and ensures you stay fuller for longer, and your metabolic health is guaranteed. Resistant starch can be found in white and brown rice, especially when you let it cool down after cooking. Keep off from refined grains as they are not a healthy choice. It also makes them have high carbohydrate levels. Unlike refined grains, whole grain can quickly turn up your metabolism.

vi. Chia Seeds

It is one of the most nutritious foods on earth. The level of fiber in chia seeds is pretty high hence making it one of the foods that have the lowest levels of carbohydrates on the surface. Chia seeds can quickly expand your stomach because of their ability to absorb up to 11 times their water weight due to the high fiber content. According to recent studies done, it was found out that chia seeds that reduce a person's appetite. Due to the type of nutrient composition in chia seeds, it makes them helpful in weight loss. When you consume chia seeds, you will be full for more extended hours.

vii. Legumes

Legumes and beans are usually low-calorie foods. Grains such as chickpeas, black beans, and kidney beans has been proven to assist in weight loss. They have very high fiber and protein content, and these are the two nutrients that enable a person to feel full for longer hours after eating. It is essential to prepare the legumes well because some people are unable to stand them, and this is because they have resistant starch.

viii. Potatoes

For optimal health, potatoes seem to have specific properties that ensure that the body is functioning well. They usually contain a very diverse range of nutrients, nearly everything needed by the body. Potassium, which is found in potatoes, has been found to play a significant role in the reduction of blood pressure. When boiled potatoes were put on a satiety index scale that measures how filling foods are, they scored the highest among all the processed foods.

What this shows is that when you eat white potatoes, you will feel fuller and have fewer cravings for other foods. A fiber-like substance that is starch resistant will be formed when you boil your vegetables and leave them to cool down. Apart from only weight loss, the fiber-like content can also lead to loss of weight.

ix. Cruciferous Veggies

When you hear about cruciferous veggies, all this means are vegetables like broccoli, cabbage, and cauliflower. These vegetables are very high in fiber and can make you full for longer hours. The other good thing about the cruciferous veggies is they contain the right amount of protein.

They do not provide high protein levels like the ones in animals or even beans, but in the vegetable kingdom, they have the highest protein levels. For weight loss, cruciferous veggies are perfect for you since they have a great combination of low energy density, proteins, and fiber. The other advantage of cruciferous vegetables are they have substances that were found to be useful in the fight against cancer. Including them in your diet will always improve your overall health.

x. Soups

For you to eat fewer calories, ensure you consume a meal that has a low energy density. Vegetables and fruits are known to have low energy densities because they contain lots of water. Studies show when you eat the same food as a soup rather than when eat it it whole, you feel fuller for longer hours at a time. It will make you eat fewer calories. When added to your soup, the cream can make you consume a lot of calories, so try and avoid it while cooking. For a weight loss diet, soup can be very filling and effective because of the water content.

Foods To Avoid

Below we shall see all the toxic foods to avoid to stay healthy during and after the fasting period.

i. Fried Foods

Fried foods usually contain calories at high levels. Most restaurants prefer deep-frying because it cuts down on costs. As much as many people love fried food, these foods are unhealthy because they contain fat. These fats are formed through a process called hydrogenation. What people who manufacture food do is they use the hydrogenation process to help the processed food last longer. During frying of foods, changes occur on their chemical structure, making it very hard for the body to break it down.

Many diseases, such as heart disease, obesity, and diabetes, are usually caused by trans-fats. Most of the time, vegetable oil is used during deep-frying, which is said to contain trans-fat even before its heated. Most people reuse frying oil, which makes the level of fats to go up even higher.

It is advisable to consume non-fried foods since they contain fewer calories. The hormones used in appetite regulation can be affected by fried foods since they lead to weight gain. Weight gain has not been associated with polyunsaturated and monounsaturated fats. People who enjoy fried foods should endeavor to prepare them in the comfort of their homes using healthy oils. Some of the healthy oils include:

- Avocado oil
- Coconut oil
- Olive oil.

Some of the health risks brought about by feeding on fried food can be minimized by using the above oils in preparing your meals. We also have oils that contain high levels of polyunsaturated fats which, when exposed to heat, will form acrylamide. Such oils should avoid at all costs when deep-frying our foods. Examples of such oils are:

- Sunflower oil
- Grapeseed oils
- Sesame oils

- Corn oil
- Canola oil
- Soybean oil.

These oils contain trans-fats even before heating them and frying your food. The bottom line is that foods cooked in unhealthy oils greatly puts your health at risk. Therefore, it is better to avoid eating foods cooked in them.

ii. Beverages Containing Sugar

Drinks that contain sugar are typically very harmful because you always take in so much that your brain will not record them as food. When we talk about beverages containing sugar, we mean sweetened coffee, sodas, milkshakes etcetera. The reason why sugary drinks are discouraged during intermittent fasting is that it leads to rapid weight gain. When you consume large amounts of sugar, it will be turned into fat by your liver hence gaining weight.

When you use large amounts of table sugar, fructose will be supplied to your body. Unlike glucose, which can be broken down by all cells in the body; it will be turned into fat. Fructose does not help you to feel full, and this may lead you to take up lots of calories. People who drink sweetened beverages are always at risk of being obese. Sugar or sweeteners are discouraged because they bring about belly fat. Belly fat, which is also known as visceral fat, can cause diabetes type 2. Sodas may cause your cells to resist insulin effects.

The carbohydrate fructose is responsible for high uric acid levels in the body. Eventually, the uric acid becomes candied, and that is when a person will start suffering from gout. When the brain is not able to function appropriately, especially in adults, they suffer from diseases such as the Alzheimer's disease. When the blood sugar levels are incredibly high, the risk of dementia also rises.

iii. Breakfast Cereals

These are grains that have gone through processing and contain high levels of added sugar. They are usually eaten with milk and are more common in children's meals. Some of the cereals are oats, rice, and even corn. Shredding and roasting are some of the processes used to ensure the breakfast cereals are a bit more edible. Most breakfast cereals have a very high sugar content. It is advisable to consume grains that have high fiber content and very minimal sugar levels.

v. White Bread

Bread has been consumed for centuries. It is made from water and flour and yeast. It is considered to be fattening, and unlike fruits and veggies, it has almost zero nutrients. Bread usually comprises of a lot of calories and carbohydrates. Eating it may not add any nutritional value to your body since it has very levels of vitamins and proteins.

Most wheat products have gluten, which is usually used to help the dough to rise before baking. Whole grain bread always has high fiber content, which will reduce the speed at which sugar will be absorbed into the bloodstream. It will then ensure the blood sugar level stabilizes.

vi. Processed Meat

Unlike its unprocessed counterpart, processed meat is very unhealthy. Studies have shown that most illnesses are caused by consuming processed meat. Heart disease, type 2 diabetes, and even colon cancer are some of the conditions that can be caused by processed meat. Processed meats have usually been conserved by canning, smoking, and even curing. Some of the processed meats include:

- Ham
- Bacon
- Salted meat
- Canned meat
- Sausages
- Salami
- Hot dogs

People who eat processed meat have been said to take meager amounts of healthy foods such as veggies and fruits. Many long-lasting illnesses nowadays have been reported to be caused by eating processed meat. Some of these illnesses include heart disease, colon cancer, and high blood pressure. It is because of the presence of chemicals they have that increases the risk of the conditions.

Processed meat has been said to contain N-nitroso compounds that are supposed to be cancer-causing. The N-nitroso compounds are made from sodium nitrite, which is used to prevent bacteria and cut food poisoning risks. It also makes the flavor better through rancidification, which means to suppress the oxidation of fat and most of all, to preserve the color of the meat, which is either red or pink.

When processed meat products are subjected to high heat, nitrosamines that play significant role illnesses such as bowel cancer forms. One of the oldest methods of meat preservation is smoking. Research shows that smoked meat can contain polycyclic aromatic hydrocarbons, also known as PAHs, which is very harmful to the body.

Another reason why it is advisable to keep away from processed meat is it contains toxic chemical compounds that form when your meat is prepared under high temperatures. These chemical compounds are known as heterocyclic amines. The research was done whereby the heterocyclic amines were given to animals, and it proved that indeed it is cancer-causing. Many studies carried out also showed than when a person frequently consumes well done red meat, they raise their chances of suffering from colon or prostate cancer.

For decades, salt has been used as a preservative, but most importantly, its work is to improve the taste of food. When you consume salt excessively, it can easily cause hypertension and other cardiovascular-related illnesses. Processed meat should also be avoided because the amount of salt that goes into their processing is high, and recent studies found out that excessive consumption of salt may cause stomach cancer.

vii. Pizza

Pizza is a food that you should stay away from when on your eating window during intermittent fasting because it has lots of calories and fat that is saturated. It usually leads to fat around the belly. Eating pizza does not add any nutritional value to the body. It only makes you have incredibly high cravings for bad carbohydrates because of getting used to eating starchy foods. When on intermittent fasting, pizza should not be eaten because when you consume lots of starch and salt, your body tends to retain water. It will make you gain more weight instead of of losing it. Overtime when you eat pizza, your, body will gain more fat.

vii. Fried Chicken

Fried chicken should be avoided like the plague during intermittent fasting. It is because apart from leading to weight gain, it can lead to significant health issues, including heart problems. A study showed that consuming fried chicken frequently was associated with many deaths, which were mainly from cardiovascular diseases and cancer. It also shows that those who regularly consume fried chicken are likely to eat fewer vegetables and other healthy foods. They will be craving for sugared beverages like soda, lots of salt, and other unprocessed meats.

The bad thing about fried chicken is it has high levels of salt, calories, and fat, which significantly affect the heart and how it functions daily. The other reason why you should avoid eating fried chicken is it contains high levels of glycation end products which can easily cause inflammation. The glycation end products are compounds usually formed when high temperatures are used for cooking.

viii. Ice Cream

Ice cream is one of the things you should stay away from when on your eating window during intermittent fasting because it has very high levels of cholesterol. The downside of the cholesterol in ice cream is it is known to increase blood cholesterol in your body. This puts you at a high risk of suffering from heart-related illnesses.

Another reason why ice cream should be avoided when doing intermittent fasting is that it contains saturated fats. Sugar is knew to be an empty calorie; therefore, it has no nutrients at all. Ice cream is one of the foods that should not be eaten because it has a lot of sugar, which will lead to weight gain and other heart diseases. When you consume sugar, it can lead to a person who has diabetes because of the quick effect it has on the levels of blood glucose.

ix. Artificial Sweeteners

When on intermittent fasting, one of the things you should highly avoid is artificial sweeteners because they lead to weight gain. Studies that were carried out showed that fake sugar caused obesity in both children and grownups. The bad thing about consuming artificial sugars is it makes your body feel like it needs more calories. That feeling will make you eat even more than you are supposed to. Some of the foods that have artificial sugars are:

- Sweetened yogurt
- Diet drinks, especially diet soda
- Protein shakes
- Baked foods and candy
- Pickles
- Salad dressings and
- Ice cream.

 People who consumer artificial sugars a lot are said to suffer from metabolic related issues such as excess belly fat, high levels of blood sugar in the body, and abnormal cholesterol levels. All this will eventually put you at a very high risk of stroke and heart disease.

When artificial sugar is taken daily, the chance of suffering from cardiovascular disease is high. Insulin is released in the body when artificial sweeteners are consumed without increasing the sugar levels in the blood. Low blood sugar will be caused due to the absorption of sugar in our bloodstream. It makes a artificial sugar consumer suffer from low levels of blood sugar, also known as hypoglycemia.

x. Chocolate

As sweet as it is, the disadvantages of eating chocolate outweigh its nutritional value making it one of the foods to avoid when on intermittent fasting. Chocolate has a very high content of saturated fats and total fats. The number of saturated fat content in chocolate is likely to increase the level of bad cholesterol in your body, putting someone at risk of suffering from heart disease. When you consume dark chocolate, it does not raise your cholesterol levels since it comes from cocoa butter. It not the same as the fat found in milk chocolate.

The other reason why during intermittent fasting you should avoid chocolate is because of the high levels of sugar in it. Both sugars in chocolate and other carbohydrates can provide energy just that they have many disadvantages. Chocolate can also cause the tooth to decay and cause heart problems due to its high sugar levels. Another reason why chocolate should be avoided is it is deficient in minerals and vitamin levels.

Drinks To Take

What To Drink While On Intermittent Fasting.

Starting any lifestyle changes takes time, and it could be confusing at the beginning. After all, you want to do it right. When it comes to intermittent fasting, one of the most common questions asked is: "What can you drink during intermittent fasting?" Staying hydrated is always essential, but it's even more so during intermittent fasting when your food intake is usually reduced. Roughly 20% of our daily water intake comes from food. Therefore, it is especially important to drink more when you are fasting. One of the side effects of intermittent fasting you might experience is a headache. While it can appear due to several reasons, dehydration is one of the most common ones.

Additionally, a bonus of drinking plenty of liquids while doing intermittent fasting – it can help to overcome the hunger during your fasting period. To get all the health benefits of Intermittent Fasting such as fat loss, increased metabolic rate, lower blood sugar levels, boost in the immune system, and others, you have to restrict from consuming any caloric food. But you can still consume non-caloric beverages because they do not break your fast and allow you to get all the benefits of fasting. This is because non-caloric beverages do not cause the release of insulin, and as a consequence, do not interfere with fat burning and autophagy (cellular cleanup).

This would include:

- Water
- Sparkling water
- Mineral water
- Plain black coffee
- Plain tea

But the question is…what exactly can you drink during intermittent fasting to not break your fast?

When fasting, you do not have to start hungry during the entire time. You can take some beverages which will not break your fast. Some of the drinks that can be taken during intermittent fasting are:

i. Coffee

Coffee has zero calories, and drinking it will not break your fast. Coffee is capable of suppressing hunger, making fasting easily doable. Black coffee cannot break your fast when you take it without milk or cream. The benefits of fasting can also be taken with coffee. Coffee and intermittent fasting can help in reducing inflammation that is chronic as this opens doors to many other diseases in the body.

One of the significant inflammation conditions characterized by high cholesterol and excess body fat is metabolic syndrome. Coffee intake usually decreases the risk of metabolic syndrome. Coffee has also been found to improve brain health just like intermittent fasting. Consistent intake of coffee has been found to reduce the risks of diseases such as Alzheimer's disease. Coffee has also been said to increase autophagy.

When on intermittent fasting, the body uses fat to produce energy, which is in the form of ketones. Like we said before, black coffee cannot make you break your fast. When you put in other additives, you are likely to break your fast and reduce the benefits of fasting. Intermittent fasting can significantly be affected by adding sugar, milk, or even cream in your coffee. Sweetened coffee that is high in calories should be avoided like the plague during the fasting window.

Examples of these types of coffee are cappuccino and lattes. When fasting, making coffee is not a must, you can either have it or not. It is a personal choice. As much as coffee does not break a fast, remember it should be taken in moderation and without any additives that have a high-calorie content.

ii. Water

Water is vital as every organ in the body uses it. It ensures that you are well-hydrated and causes the body not to feel any hunger. Water is a essential drink because apart from making sure you have a regular digestive system, it also ensures that your joints are lubricated and you have a well-regulated body temperature.

Research shows water can also help you burn more calories. When the amount of calories you use up increases, it is called resting energy expenditure. Studies show that, in obese children, the resting energy expenditure increased significantly due to drinking enough water. Studies done on overweight adults showed that drinking 1.5 liters of water daily for a few weeks led to a reduction of fat around the abdomen, weight, and body mass index.

Another reason why water is encouraged during intermittent fasting is that it curbs appetite and helps you to eat moderately, but still feel full.

Thorough research was carried out on adults, and it showed that drinking water before having your meals could cause a person to lose up to 2 kilograms over 12 weeks. Just by drinking water in the morning before having your breakfast, you can significantly reduce the number of calories in that meal by nearly 15%.

Water is said to reduce weight since it has zero calories. Parents are also advised to encourage their children to drink water as this will reduce the risk of obesity. It is said that the amount of water intake per day should be 2 liters. Very sporty people who do lots of exercises may need more water than those who are less active.

Water can be found in other foods and drinks as well, such as in vegetables, milk, fish, tea, and even fruits. Drinking water through your fasting windows when on intermittent fasting may help you to reduce hunger, headaches, and even prevent someone from having a bad mood. This is because the above symptoms may be caused by mild dehydration. You should also be warned that drinking too much water may cause water toxicity, which is not suitable for your health.

iii. Green Tea

Green tea is said to be one of the healthiest beverages. The antioxidants present in green tea are very advantageous to the body. People who are on intermittent fasting are encouraged to drink green tea during the fasting window. It dramatically improves the rate at which fat is lost and also helps increase brain activity. Green tea is supported since when you take it, you are guaranteed of improved physical performance.

The metabolic rate is also one of the significant improvements which occur by drinking green tea. Two studies that were carried out with male adults showed that after taking green tea, the rate at which fat was oxidized was increased by almost 20%. The energy expenditure was also increased.

It has also been proven that green tea can protect your brain from diseases such as Alzheimer's and Parkinson's disease. This is possible because it protects your mind for both the short and long term due to the catechin compounds found in green tea that protects neurons in the brain. It will, in turn, protect the brain from neurodegenerative illnesses that leads to Parkinson's disease.

Green tea is usually used during intermittent fasting because it has bioactive compounds that are known to improve health. Green tea can also help in the fight against cancer due to the presence of polyphenols, which are very useful in the reduction of inflammation. The catechin, which is also present in green tea helps in the prevention of cell damage. The benefits of green tea are so many. That is why it is advisable to drink it during your fasting period. Another thing is it helps reduce the risk of cancers, such as:

- Colorectal cancer
- Prostate cancer
- Breast cancer.

Another reason why green tea is essential is that it lowers your risk of infection by killing bacteria. It also helps people to avoid cavities in their teeth by killing the harmful bacteria found in the mouth, which is known as streptococcus. It is advisable to drink green tea during your fasting window due to its benefit of lowering the risk of diabetes type 2. Just by taking green tea, insulin sensitivity can be significantly reduced and thus reducing the blood sugar levels.

Green tea has also been proven to reduce the risk of cardiovascular illnesses. It can also increase the capacity of antioxidants in the blood that prevent the oxidation of LDL. The best benefit of green tea is that it helps in weight loss by boosting the metabolic rate, which eventually decreases body fat. It has also been proven to cause longevity. It is because when you drink it, it lowers your risk of heart disease and cancer that can cut short your life.

To become smarter than you are already, all you need is to drink green tea. The key active ingredient is caffeine that blocks the adenosine. It is an inhibitory transmitter of the neurons. From the studies carried out on caffeine, it has been proven that caffeine can improve memory, vigilance, and causs someone to have good moods all day.

Iv. Chicken Broth

When chicken broth is cooked correctly, it will release nutrients such as magnesium, collagen, gelatin, and calcium. Chicken broth is one of the most amazing foods because even during sickness, it can make you feel better as is a health-boosting drink. It is advisable to drink chicken broth when on intermittent fasting as it helps in reducing inflammation, increases immunity, and protect your gut as well.

The reason for eating chicken broth during intermittent fasting is because it has the amino acid known as glycine that can boost anti-inflammatory. The glycine is also essential as it helps in detoxification, which eventually burns fat. The other importance of chicken broth is that it can drastically improve both the repair and growth of bones. This is thanks to the many minerals present in the chicken broth such as phosphorus, calcium, and magnesium.

V. Herbal Tea

Herbs, flowers, and roots are some of the ingredients used in making herbal tea. Herbal tea usually has lots of medicinal values which range from relieving stress to treating a cold. Herbal tea can be taken to boost immunity. It is possible because of the presence of vitamins and antioxidants that help in the fight against diseases and infections.

Another reason why herbal tea is useful when on the intermittent fasting journey is because it will lower your blood pressure, especially hibiscus tea. Herbal tea can also be helpful to people who find it hard to sleep. They can benefit from the herbal tea as it calms the mind when taken just before going to bed. One of the herbal teas that reduce stress and anxiety is chamomile tea. It is most comforting as well and might cause mild stimulation in the brain to reduce the feeling of depression.

Herbal tea is essential because it has a anti-aging effect. They have antioxidants which research has shown slows down the aging process by reducing the aging of the body cells and preventing them from getting damaged. The herbal tea will make you look and even feel younger, and it will genuinely show on your face and hair.

Herbal tea has also been found to improve digestion. Indigestion, bloating, and even vomiting are some of the symptoms that can be cured by taking herbal tea because they cause the breakdown of fat and rapid emptying of the stomach. When you consume herbal tea, it will keep you from needing to take medicines. For issues like treating cold, it has properties that help in clearing the nasal passage and stops heavy coughs.

Vi. Apple Juice

During intermittent fasting, apple juice is one of the essential fluids you can take during your eating window. This is an essential benefit of apple juice because this build-up may lead to a stroke. The antioxidant boost when apple juice is taken means that the heart is protected against diseases. When on intermittent fasting, apple juice taken during the eating window can be beneficial in that it contains 88% water hence very healthy.

The liquid is much recommended because it can cause hydration very quickly. It is even better for sick children because they can consume it quickly due to its great taste and the fact that it can speedily hydrate them. Extensive research was carried out, and it showed that children who were suffering from diarrhea and vomiting did not need fluids delivered via their veins, unlike those that were given electrolytes.

Apple juice has also been found to be very important, especially as age starts to catch up with you as it will support mental health. Unstable molecules in your brain known as free molecules may cause damages, causing the mind not to function at its optimum level. Apple juice will protect the brain thanks to the polyphenols and antioxidant activity found in the apple juice.

vii. Soymilk

Soymilk is a nondairy product made from soybeans. Most people, who do not drink dairy milk, usually prefer soy milk because milk from cows contains sugars known as lactose, and some people may have trouble digesting it. Soymilk is packed with all the essential amino acids which have many health benefits. It also has the right balance of carbohydrates and fats as well as very high protein levels. Soy milk also has less saturated fat, and this will ensure you do not add weight from it, especially when on intermittent fasting. Soy milk has a protective value against heart problems.

vii. Sea Saltwater

When fasting, most nutrients, and minerals in your body get depleted fast. That is why it is the importance of having sodium in your meals to help you stay hydrated because the muscle cells will be able to take in water. For it to work effectively, a person is allowed to add half a teaspoon of sea salt to four liters of water.

viii. Apple Cider Vinegar

Apple cider is famous during intermittent fasting because it assists the body in the absorption of nutrients and balancing of sugar levels thanks to acetic acid. People with type 2 diabetes or insulin resistance can significantly benefit from apple cider vinegar as it will help your blood sugar levels stay healthy. The vinegar will lower blood sugar levels and ensure insulin sensitivity is improved. Another benefit apple cider vinegar is the quick absorption of minerals from food. Apple cider vinegar is essential when fasting because it suppresses the appetite. It is advisable to take apple cider vinegar due to its capability to curb hunger.

ix. Carbonated Water

When carbon dioxide gas is infused with water under pressure, it becomes carbonated water, which is also known as carbonated water. , sodium chloride and other minerals are sometimes added and small amounts to improve the water taste. When a chemical reaction occurs between carbon dioxide and water, carbonic acid is produced. This will help maintain the blood alkalinity.

Unlike plain water, when taken, carbonated water may make someone feel fuller for longer hours, and that is why it is recommended during intermittent fasting. Some studies found that carbonated water reduced the chances of constipation. Carbonated or club soda water can improve heart health by decreasing the levels of bad cholesterol. When the water was consumed, it also increased the level of good cholesterol.

Advantages Of Intermittent Fasting

I. Promoting Health & Weight Loss

Results in several human studies have found that alternate-day and whole-day Intermittent Fasting has been associated with a significant decrease in body weight, body fat, and waist circumference both short and long term, but has also been frequently observed in some time-restricted Intermittent Fasting studies.

In an early 2019 systematic review, all of the studies reviewed experienced weight loss. However, they noted individuals tended to lose MORE weight earlier on in the study compared to the final follow-up point. This likely due to the study's dropout rates.

On top of that, in a more recent 2019 systematic review and meta-analysis, weekly Intermittent Fasting interventions were just as effective as Continuous Energy Restriction (CER) for weight loss. This proved it was not necessary to starve yourself every single day. With a more flexible diet like Intermittent Fasting, you could yield the same weight loss results. One thing to keep in mind is that many of these studies are short-term so it's unclear whether they could keep the weight off.

ii. Intermittent Fasting Promotes Improved Body Composition

When you're fasting, you're not consuming calories, so it makes sense to assume that with eating less than you normally would, you're going to lose weight. Fasting allows you to use up all of your stored sugars as fuel, and to then tap into fat stores. When we begin to burn fat stores, we begin to lose body fat. Intermittent fasting helps to improve body composition by demanding a caloric deficit, promoting weight loss and decreased body fat and causing positive changes to our metabolism via its effects on hormones.

iii. Reduces Fat-Free Mass

Diets that continually restrict calories, reduce body fat, but also Fat-Free Mass (FFM). Fat-Free Mass is everything other than fat. This is no good because that means you are losing lean muscle mass. However, studies have shown that with sufficient protein intake and resistance training, Intermittent Fasting may help to retain lose fat mass while retaining more of their lean mass (aka. our fat-burning lean muscle!) compared to daily calorie restriction-type of diets.

iv. Bravo To Increased Brain Functioning

This is one of the common benefits of intermittent fasting. Studies have explored the powerful effects of this time-restricted diet on cognitive performance (such as memory). IF is beneficial especially for athletes whether they are exercising or at rest (here, here). A 2018 systematic review found that weight loss, in general, is associated with improvements in cognitive function.

v. It's Simple

This eating pattern is easily implemented and for those who like routine, it can be adhered to fairly easily. For some people, it may be easy to incorporate into your current routine. For example, did you know that the common "Time-restricted feeding" type of Intermittent Fasting is often unintentionally practiced by those who skip breakfast and do not eat after an early dinner each day.

vi. It's Easier To Follow

Research has found people find it easier to follow a intermittent fasting diet over a long-term period compared to following a calorie-restricted diet. It is suggested that as individuals only have to reduce their calorie intake every other day on the ADF diet, it is easier to achieve than lowering consumption every day. Even those who follow the amended ADF diet, where they can consume 500 calories on "fast days," have found that much more achievable than maintaining a constant calorie deficit. Therefore, for those wanting to achieve sustainable weight loss, intermittent fasting might be extremely beneficial.

vii. Aids Digestion

Intermittent Fasting can positively impact the microbiome (our colony of gut bacteria that is essential to good digestion, mood, and immunity), as well as strengthen our intestinal barrier and help support the gut's natural circadian rhythm. As a culture, we have a habit of constantly eating and snacking - and this puts constant pressure on our digestive tract. A period of fasting helps our bodies complete their digestive processes and gives us a rest, especially in the evening when metabolism may be slower.

viii. Reduced Blood Pressure

IF may help lower high blood pressure in the short term. A study published in June 2018 in Nutrition and Healthy Aging found 16:8 significantly decreased the systolic blood pressure among the 23 study participants. The link has been shown in both animal and human studies, according to to a review published in March 2019 in Nutrients. And, an October 2019 study published in the European Journal of

Nutrition found IF led to even greater reductions in systolic blood pressure than another diet that did not involve defined eating times.

Having a healthy blood pressure is important as unhealthy levels can increase your risk for heart disease, stroke, and kidney disease. But so far the research shows these blood pressure benefits last only while IF is practiced. Once the diet ended and people returned to eating as normal, researchers found the blood pressure readings returned to their initial levels.

ix. No Macronutrient Limitations

There are popular eating plans that significantly restrict specific macronutrients. For example, many people follow a low-carb eating plan to boost health or lose weight. Others follow a low-fat diet for medical or weight-loss purposes. Each of these programs requires the consumer to adopt a new way of eating often replacing favorite foods with new and possibly unfamiliar foods. This may require new cooking skills and learning to shop and stock the kitchen differently. None of these skills are required when intermittent fasting simply because their is no target macronutrient range and no macronutrients are restricted or forbidden.

x. Reduces Inflammation Throughout Your Body

Inflammation is bad because it causes stress to your body and causes damage to cells. Things like high blood sugar, smoking, and being sick will cause your body to be in a state of inflammation. One of the bad side effects of inflammation is that your body will not be wanting to use fat as energy. Our blood sugar remains high and insulin is elevated in response. This is an anti-inflammatory lifestyle, on top of that the clean foods like whole grains and vegetables that you will be eating are anti-inflammatory foods.

Disadvantages Of Intermittent Fasting

I. It Can Be Hard To Stick With Long-Term

Intermittent fasting requires that you go a designated period without eating at all, then you eat a designated amount of calories in a specific window of time, and repeat to create a caloric deficit. This prolonged period of zero-calorie consumption can be difficult to stick with long-term due to low energy, cravings, habits, and the discipline required to stick to the specific time frames surrounding your periods of intermittent fasting. Intermittent fasting is also hard to stick with long-term due to the amount of self-control required to do so. Both sides of intermittent fasting can be difficult; not eating when you're supposed to be fasting, and not bingeing when it's time to eat are equally important.

ii. Interference With The Social Aspect Of Eating

Eating is very much a social activity. When you think about it, all of our celebrations, milestones and special occasions revolve around food. This new style of eating is very different from the typical daily eating patterns of most people. This is because of the shortened timeframe you have for eating. It can be difficult for you in social gatherings where everyone else is eating and sipping on beverages, making you awkwardly stand out from the crowd. Not to mention, you might be missing out on those late-night romantic dinners, home-made family suppers, birthday dinners, lunch meetings with your boss, and co-workers, and maybe even sharing a meal with your spouse and kids. Not so fun.

iii. The First Few Weeks Are The Hardest

Like with any good thing, fasting does have its downsides. Once you start fasting the first few weeks to a month will be the hardest. If you're used to eating constantly throughout the day and then stop, your body will freak out a bit. During this transition period, you must take it easy on yourself. Going from eating all day to once a day is probably not the best approach.

I suggest you:

- Start with the 16/8 protocol- As I mentioned earlier.
- Drink lots of water while fasting- Water will help with hunger. Adding a bit of sea salt will also help you flush out toxins.
- Break you're fast if you feel dizzy or sick. Even if you fast for 12–14 hours that's a great start. You can work your way up to longer fasting periods gradually.
- Make sure you are eating a proper amount of calories- It's easy to go into an extreme caloric deficit with intermittent fasting. Make sure your meals are filling and nutritious.

iv. Digestion Issues

Some of us may experience digestion problems when they eat large amounts of food in a short amount of time. Larger volumes of food translates to more time needed to digest. This can cause additional stress on your GI tract, leading to indigestion and bloating. This can have huge implications for those with IBS. They already have a more sensitive gut, inflammation of the GI, and disturbed bowel movements. Therefore they are more susceptible to cramping, abdominal pain and bloating. Especially with IBS, you may already have difficulty obtaining all your nutritional requirements due to the uncomfortable symptoms that come along with it. That's why people with digestive issues are recommended to eat at regular times, take time when eating, and not skip meals so as to have regular bowel functions.

v. Difficult Adjustment Period

Aside from possibly having to skip out on brunch with your friends or snack time with the coworkers, there are a few other changes that may require time to adjust to. Due to their fixation on food, many people will find themselves constantly obsessing overeating while fasting. Subsequently, you may experience low energy levels, difficulty focusing, heartburn, and headaches which can affect your mood and productivity. However, it is important to note that these symptoms subside after about a week or two, and your desire for food will lessen over time. So if you can stand it, hang in there!

vi. It Isn't For Everyone!

If you have a medical condition, it is best to avoid this type of fasting. For instance, individuals with diabetes or hypoglycemia need glucose throughout the day and going without can have dangerous effects. If you are one of those people who feel nauseous or just don't feel great going too long without eating, Intermittent Fasting may not suitable for you. It's also important to note that if you have ever had a history of an eating disorder, Intermittent Fasting is not for you.

Since Intermittent Fasting causes you to eat more food in a short amount of time, it may exacerbate potential disordered eating patterns such as a "binge-eating" mentality. This could cause you to eat more food than your body can handle, or a "restrictive" mindset to become skinnier. This will have adverse effects on your relationship with food and your body's physical health

vii. Slower Metabolism

Rather than overeating, Intermittent Fasting can make you have a slower metabolism as your body goes into starvation mode and begins to use your muscle protein as a source of fuel. Even a short 24-hour fast can lower your BMR (Basal Metabolic Rate), having negative health implications in the long run! For many of us, a better weight-loss approach may be eating several small meals throughout the day. This stabilizes our insulin levels and blood glucose. It also prevents any sort of ravenous meal gorging at the end of the day. Eating 6 times a day may help maintain your lean muscle mass (which means faster metabolism!) compared to eating less frequently.

viii. Slower Detoxing

In comparison to liquid fasting and other experimental fasting techniques, Intermittent Fasting is a slower detoxing process because one is generally still eating foods and digesting. This means that in an overall sense, Intermittent fasting will not yield the same results as a 30-day liquid cleanse will do. This is very important when considering getting into this. I would say from personal experience that a period of 4 months of Intermittent fasting is more or less equal to a month of liquid fasting. It's a great comparison in terms of seeing the detoxing power of fasting as a whole.

ix. Overeating, Lethargy

Another important factor associated with the harmful effects of intermittent fasting is the appetite not being effectively satisfied. Although a person is physically full, he/she will be tempted to eat more. This behavior leads to over-eating, and it almost kills the underlying purpose of losing weight by starting intermittent fasting in the first place. Another chapter of this unfortunate dark side of intermittent fasting is the (reportedly) drastically reduced energy levels during the earlier parts of the day. This results in a person feeling lazy and lethargic during work and also causes reduced concentration levels that can affect one's ability to carry out day to day activities.

x. Increased Hunger

A regular side-effect of fasting diets is that they can alter the balance of your hormones. Specifically, the reduction in leptin (which makes you feel full), and the increase in cortisol (which can result in your body being under more stress, and thus a halt in weight loss). A University of Virginia Study on fasting showed female students' leptin decreased by as much as 75% and their cortisol increased by as much as 50% after the fasting period of the study. Increased cortisol can also result in changes in the menstrual cycle for women.

CHAPTER 5: THE KETO DIET AND INTERMITTENT FASTING

What Is Ketogenic Diet ?

The ketogenic diet is a very low-carb, high-fat diet that shares many similarities with the Atkins and low-carb diets. It involves drastically reducing carbohydrate intake and replacing it with fat. This reduction in carbs puts your body into a metabolic state called ketosis. When this happens, your body becomes incredibly efficient at burning fat for energy. It also turns fat into ketones in the liver, which can supply energy for the brain.

The Keto diet involves going long spells on extremely low (no higher than 30g per day) to almost zero g per day of carbs and increasing your fats to a high level (to the point where they may make up as much as 65% of your daily macronutrients intake.) The idea behind this is to get your body into a state of ketosis. In this state of ketosis, the body is supposed to be more inclined to use fat for energy- and research says it does just this. Depleting your carbohydrate/glycogen liver stores and then moving onto fat for fuel means you should end up being shredded.

Different Types Of Ketogenic Diets

There Are Several Versions Of The Ketogenic Diet, Including:

- The standard ketogenic diet (SKD): This is a very low-carb, moderate-protein and high-fat diet. It typically contains 75% fat, 20% protein and only 5% carbs (1Trusted Source).

- The cyclical ketogenic diet (CKD): This diet involves periods of higher-carb refeeds, such as 5 ketogenic days followed by 2 high-carb days.
- The targeted ketogenic diet (TKD): This diet allows you to add carbs around workouts.
- High-protein ketogenic diet: This is similar to a standard ketogenic diet, but includes more protein. The ratio is often 60% fat, 35% protein, and 5% carbs.

A Sample Keto Meal Plan For 1 Week

To help get you started, here is a sample ketogenic diet meal plan for one week:

Monday

- Breakfast: Bacon, eggs, and tomatoes.
- Lunch: Chicken salad with olive oil and feta cheese.
- Dinner: Salmon with asparagus cooked in butter.

Tuesday

- Breakfast: Egg, tomato, basil, and goat cheese omelet.
- Lunch: Almond milk, peanut butter, cocoa powder, and stevia milkshake.
- Dinner: Meatballs, cheddar cheese, and vegetables.

Wednesday

- Breakfast: A ketogenic milkshake (try this or this).
- Lunch: Shrimp salad with olive oil and avocado.
- Dinner: Pork chops with Parmesan cheese, broccoli, and salad.

Thursday

- Breakfast: Omelet with avocado, salsa, peppers, onion, and spices.

- Lunch: A handful of nuts and celery sticks with guacamole and salsa.
- Dinner: Chicken stuffed with pesto and cream cheese, along with vegetables.

Friday

- Breakfast: Sugar-free yogurt with peanut butter, cocoa powder, and stevia.
- Lunch: Beef stir-fry cooked in coconut oil with vegetables.
- Dinner: Bun-less burger with bacon, egg, and cheese.

Saturday

- Breakfast: Ham and cheese omelet with vegetables.
- Lunch: Ham and cheese slices with nuts.
- Dinner: Whitefish, egg, and spinach cooked in coconut oil.

Sunday

- Breakfast: Fried eggs with bacon and mushrooms.
- Lunch: Burger with salsa, cheese, and guacamole.
- Dinner: Steak and eggs with a side salad.

Always try to rotate the vegetables and meat over the long-term, as each type provides different nutrients and health benefits.

Supplements For A Ketogenic Diet

Although no supplements are required, some can be useful.

- MCT oil: Added to drinks or yogurt, MCT oil provides energy and helps increase ketone levels. Take a look at several options on Amazon.
- Minerals: Added salt and other minerals can be important when starting due to shifts in water and mineral balance.

- Caffeine: Caffeine can have benefits for energy, fat loss, and performance.
- Exogenous ketones: This supplement may help raise the body's ketone levels.
- Creatine: Creatine provides numerous benefits for health and performance. This can help if you are combining a ketogenic diet with exercise.
- Whey: Use half a scoop of whey protein in shakes or yogurt to increase your daily protein intake.

Healthy Keto Snacks

In case you get hungry between meals, here are some healthy, keto-approved snacks:

- Fatty meat or fish
- Cheese
- A handful of nuts or seeds
- Cheese with olives
- 1–2 hard-boiled eggs
- 90% dark chocolate
- A low-carb milkshake with almond milk, cocoa powder, and nut butter
- Full-fat yogurt mixed with nut butter and cocoa powder
- Strawberries and cream
- Celery with salsa and guacamole
- Smaller portions of leftover meals

Tips For Eating Out On A Ketogenic Diet

- It is not very hard to make most restaurant meals keto-friendly when eating out.
- Most restaurants offer some kind of meat or fish-based dish. Order this, and replace any high-carb food with extra vegetables.

- Egg-based meals are also a great option, such as an omelet or eggs and bacon.
- Another favorite is bun-less burgers. You could also swap the fries for vegetables instead. Add extra avocado, cheese, bacon or eggs.
- At Mexican restaurants, you can enjoy any type of meat with extra cheese, guacamole, salsa, and sour cream.
- For dessert, ask for a mixed cheese board or berries with cream.

Side Effects And How To Minimize Them

Although the ketogenic diet is safe for healthy people, there may be some initial side effects while your body adapts. This is often referred to as the keto flu and is usually over within a few days.

Keto flu includes poor energy and mental function, increased hunger, sleep issues, nausea, digestive discomfort and decreased exercise performance. To minimize this, you can try a regular low-carb diet for the first few weeks. This may teach your body to burn more fat before you eliminate carbs.

A ketogenic diet can also change the water and mineral balance of your body, so adding extra salt to your meals or taking mineral supplements can help. For minerals, try taking 3,000–4,000 mg of sodium, 1,000 mg of potassium and 300 mg of magnesium per day to minimize side effects. At least, in the beginning, it is important to eat until you're full and avoid restricting calories too much. Usually, a ketogenic diet causes weight loss without intentional calorie restriction.

A Ketogenic Diet Is Great, but Not for Everyone

A ketogenic diet can be great for people who are overweight, diabetic or looking to improve their metabolic health. It may be less suitable for elite athletes or those wishing to add large amounts of muscle or weight.

And, as with any diet, it will only work if you are consistent and stick with it in the long term. That being said, few things are as well proven in nutrition as the powerful health and weight loss benefits of a ketogenic diet.

Uses And Benefits Of The Ketogenic Diet

When using a ketogenic diet, your body becomes more of a fat-burner than a carbohydrate-dependent machine. Several kinds of research have linked the consumption of increased amounts of carbohydrates to the development of several disorders such as diabetes and insulin resistance. By nature, carbohydrates are easily absorbable and therefore can also be easily stored by the body. Digestion of carbohydrates starts right from the moment you put them into your mouth. As soon as you begin chewing them, amylase (the enzymes that digest carbohydrate) in your saliva is already at work acting on carbohydrate-containing food.

In the stomach, carbohydrates are further broken down. When they get into the small intestines, they are then absorbed into the bloodstream. On getting to the bloodstream, carbohydrates generally increase the blood sugar level. This increase in blood sugar levels stimulates the immediate release of insulin into the bloodstream. The higher the increase in blood sugar levels, the more the amount of insulin that is released.

Insulin is a hormone that causes excess sugar in the bloodstream to be removed to lower the blood sugar level. Insulin takes the sugar and carbohydrate that you eat and stores them either as glycogen in muscle tissues or as fat in adipose tissue for future use as energy.

However, the body can develop what is known as insulin resistance when it is continuously exposed to such high amounts of glucose in the bloodstream. This scenario can easily cause obesity as the body tends to quickly store any excess amount of glucose. Health conditions such as diabetes and cardiovascular disease can also result from this condition. Keto diets are low in carbohydrates and high in fat and have been associated with reducing and improving several health conditions.

One of the foremost things a ketogenic diet does is to stabilize your insulin levels and also restore leptin signaling. Reduced amounts of insulin in the bloodstream allow you to feel fuller for a longer period and also to have fewer cravings.

Medical Benefits Of Ketogenic Diets

The application and implementation of the ketogenic diet have expanded considerably. Keto diets are often indicated as part of the treatment plan in several medical conditions.

Epilepsy

This is the main reason for the development of the ketogenic diet. For some reason, the rate of epileptic seizures reduces when patients are placed on a keto diet. Pediatric epileptic cases are the most responsive to the keto diet. Some children have experienced seizure elimination after a few years of using a keto diet. Children with epilepsy are generally expected to fast for a few days before starting the ketogenic diet as part of their treatment.

Cancer

Research suggests that the therapeutic efficacy of the ketogenic diets against tumor growth can be enhanced when combined with certain drugs and procedures under a "press-pulse" paradigm. It is also promising to note that ketogenic diets drive the cancer cell into remission. This means that keto diets "starve cancer" to reduce the symptoms.

Alzheimer's Disease

There are several indications that the memory functions of patients with Alzheimer's disease improve after making use of a ketogenic diet. Ketones are a great source of alternative energy for the brain especially when it has become resistant to insulin. Ketones also provide substrates (cholesterol) that help to repair damaged neurons and membranes.

These all help to improve memory and cognition in Alzheimer's patients.

Diabetes

It is generally agreed that carbohydrates are the main culprit in diabetes. Therefore, by reducing the amount of ingested carbohydrate by using a ketogenic diet, there are increased chances for improved blood sugar control. Also, combining a keto diet with other diabetes treatment plans can significantly improve their overall effectiveness.

Gluten Allergy

Many individuals with a gluten allergy are undiagnosed with this condition. However, following a ketogenic diet showed improvement in related symptoms like digestive discomforts and bloating. Most carbohydrate-rich foods are high in gluten. Thus, by using a keto diet, a lot of gluten consumption is reduced to a minimum due to the elimination of a large variety of carbohydrates.

Weight Loss

This is arguably the most common "intentional" use of the ketogenic diet today. It has found a niche for itself in the mainstream dieting trend. Keto diets have become part of many dieting regimens due to its well-acknowledged side effect of aiding weight loss. Though initially maligned by many, the growing number of favorable weight loss results has helped the ketogenic to better embraced as a major weight loss program. Besides the above medical benefits, ketogenic diets also provide some general health benefits which include the following.

Improved Insulin Sensitivity

This is the first aim of a ketogenic diet. It helps to stabilize your insulin levels thereby improving fat burning.

Muscle Preservation

Since protein is oxidized, it helps to preserve lean muscle. Losing lean muscle mass causes an individual's metabolism to slow down as muscles are generally very metabolic. Using a keto diet helps to preserve your muscles while your body burns fat.

Controlled Ph And Respiratory Function

A keto diet helps to decrease lactate thereby improving both pH and respiratory function. A state of ketosis, therefore, helps to keep your blood pH at a healthy level.

Improved Immune System

Using a ketogenic diet helps to fight off aging antioxidants while also reducing inflammation of the gut, thereby making your immune system stronger.

Reduced Cholesterol Levels

Consuming fewer carbohydrates while you are on the keto diet will help to reduce blood cholesterol levels. This is due to the increased state of lipolysis. This leads to a reduction in LDL cholesterol levels and an increase in HDL cholesterol levels.

Reduced Appetite and Cravings

Adopting a ketogenic diet helps you to reduce both your appetite and cravings for calorie-rich foods. As you begin eating healthy, satisfying, and beneficial high-fat foods, your hunger feelings will naturally start decreasing.

Tips for Exercising When on a Ketogenic Diet

A lot of things happen when you are exercising. Some of these are good for your health and others are not so good - like when you exercise excessively.

Exercise is a stressor. While it can be a good stressor, it can, however, cause your adrenals to go into overdrive. This situation increases your insulin levels and therefore reduces your ability to lose weight. When exercising, your insulin levels go up while your hunger reduces. However, this often results in a significant reduction in blood sugar levels which results in you becoming hungrier.

However, if your body is fueled with carbs, you will mostly be burning glucose for energy. This makes it a lot difficult for your body to burn and lose body fat. It is, however, important to understand that while exercise can help you lose weight, it is more important to get the diet right first. When you get the diet right, such a by using a well-designed ketogenic diet, your body will start tapping into its fat deposits for generating its energy. This is what effectively enables you to start burning and losing body fat.

Once your body gets used to the ketogenic diet, you will start feeling more energetic. At such a point, you will be better positioned to adjust your menus to start building strength and muscles. When you get to this point during the "standard ketogenic" diet, you can then alter the diet to either a "targeted" or a "cyclical" ketogenic diet. These versions of the ketogenic diet allow more carbohydrate consumption to enable you to engage in more exercise for longer.

Targeted Ketogenic Diet

The Targeted Ketogenic Diet allows you to ingest more carbs around your exercise period. This form of the diet allows you to engage in high-intensity exercise while remaining in ketosis. The carb intake within this window provides your muscles with the necessary glucose to effectively engage in your workouts. The extra glucose should normally be used up during this window of about 30 minutes and should not affect your overall metabolism.

The Targeted Ketogenic Diet is designed for beginners or intermittent exercisers. The TKD allows a slight increase in your carb consumption. However, it does not kick you out ketosis and causes no shock to your system.

Cyclical Ketogenic Diet

The Cyclical Ketogenic Diet is more appropriate for advanced athletes and bodybuilders. It is generally used for maximum muscle-building results. There is however a strong tendency for other individuals to end up adding some body fat. This is because it is easy to overeat while using the Cyclical Ketogenic Diet (CKD).

In this version of the ketogenic diet, the individual follows the standard ketogenic diet for 5 or 6 days. He or she is then allowed to eat increased amounts of carbohydrates for 1 or 2 days. As a caution, it can take a beginner close to 3 weeks to fully get back into ketosis if he or she attempts the CKD. It requires real commitment and advanced exercise levels to successfully carry out a CKD.

The Cyclical Ketogenic Diet aims to temporarily switch out of ketosis. This window allows the body to refill the amount of glycogen in the muscles to enable it to undertake the next cycle of intense workouts.

Therefore, there must be a complete depletion of the resultant glycogen build up during the subsequent workouts to get back into ketosis. The intensity of your planned workout will consequently determine the amount of increased carbohydrate intake.

Cardio Exercises

When you exercise at an intense rate, a lot of amazing things happen to your body. When you engage in cardiovascular exercises, they help to improve the efficiency of your heart and lungs. This also helps to increase the rate at which your body burns energy and over time this will lead to weight loss.

Engaging in cardio exercise causes many metabolic changes that positively affect fat metabolism. Cardiovascular exercises help to increase oxygen delivery through improved blood flow. This way, body cells can more effectively oxidize and burn fat.

This also has the effect of increasing the number of oxidative enzymes. Consequently, the speed at which fatty acids are transported to the mitochondria to be burned for energy is greatly increased.

During cardio exercises, the sensitivity of muscles and fat cells to epinephrine is greatly increased. This increases the number of triglycerides released into the blood and muscles to be burned for energy.

Strength Training

Strength training helps to improve your moods while also helping to build healthy bones. It also helps you to develop an overall strong and healthy body. Using a well-designed ketogenic will help you preserve your muscles even when carrying our strength training. Muscles are built with protein and not fat or carbs. Also, given the fact that protein oxidation is less in a ketogenic diet, engaging in strength training should not be a problem. You need to challenge your body with heavyweights to see results and get a stronger body.

Interval Training

Interval training is simply alternating intervals of high-intensity and low-intensity workouts. It is simply for you to: go fast, go slow, and repeat. While sounding so simple, interval training is one of the most powerful ways to burn body fat quickly. Apart from burning fat while carrying out interval training, the "afterburn effect" stimulates your metabolism for a longer period.

Circuit Training: Cardio + Strength

Circuit training is the combining of cardiovascular exercises with strength training exercises. This combination helps to provide all-over fitness benefits. This form of exercising combines cardio exercises such as jogging and a resistance workout without allowing a resting period between them. The lack of rest in-between both exercises makes circuit training as effective as a cardio-based high-intensity interval training workout.

Yoga

The exercise benefits of yoga come from its ability to help the body reduce levels of stress hormones and also increase insulin sensitivity. Yoga helps you to consciously connect with your body. This connection can translate into you being more mindful of how your body works and changing even your eating habits.

Why The Keto Diet Is So Effective for People Over 50

The keto diet has gained popularity in recent years and has become a nutritional plan favored by individuals of all ages. That said, this dietary roadmap might precipitate particularly important health benefits to persons over age 50.

Keto Diet Overview

Scientifically classified the ketogenic diet, this nutritional plan stresses the decreased consumption of foods containing carbohydrates and an increased intake of fats. The reduced intake of carbohydrates is said to eventually place the bodies of participating dieters into a biological and metabolic process known as ketosis.

Once ketosis is established, medical researchers opine the body becomes especially efficient in burning fat and turning said substances into energy. Moreover, during this process, the body is thought to metabolize fat into chemicals categorized as ketones, which are also said to provide significant energy sources.

[An accelerator of this is an intermittent fasting method where the restricting of carbs causes your body to access the next available energy source or ketones that are derived from stored fat. In this absence of glucose, fat is now burned by the body for energy.]

There Are Several Other Specific Ketogenic Diets Including:

Targeted (TKD)

Those participating in this version gradually add small amounts of carbohydrates into their diet.

Cyclical (CKD)

Adherents to this dietary plan consume carbohydrates on a cyclical basis like every few days or weeks.

High-Protein

High-protein diet observers consume greater quantities of protein as part of their dietary plans.

Standard (SKD)

Typically, this most commonly practiced version of the diet intake significantly diminished concentrations of carbohydrates (perhaps as little as five percent of all dietary consumption), along with protein-laden foods and a high quantity of fat products (in some cases, as much as 75 percent of all dietary needs).

Recommended Foods

Keto diet adherents are encouraged to consume foods like meat, fatty fishes, dairy products such as cheeses, milk, butter and cream, eggs, produce products possessing low carbohydrate concentrations, condiments like salt, pepper and a host of other spices, various needs, and seeds and oils like olive and coconut. On the other hand, certain foods should be avoided or strictly limited. Said items include beans and legumes, many fruits, edibles with high sugar contents, alcohol and grain products.

Keto Diet Benefits To Individuals Over 50

Keto diet adherents, especially those aged 50 and older, are said to enjoy numerous potential health benefits including:

Increased Physical And Mental Energy

As people grow older, energy levels might drop for a variety of biological and environmental reasons. Keto diet adherents often witness a boost in strength and vitality. One reason said occurrence happens is because the body is burning excess fat, which in turn gets synthesized into energy. Furthermore, systemic synthesis of ketones tends to increase brain power and stimulate cognitive functions like focus and memory.

Improved Sleep

Individuals tend to sleep less as they age. Keto dieters often gain more from exercise programs and become tired easier. Said occurrence could precipitate longer and more fruitful periods of rest.

Metabolism

Aging individuals often experience a slower metabolism than they did during their younger days. Long-time keto dieters experience a greater regulation of blood sugar, which can increase their metabolic rates.

Weight Loss

Faster and more efficient metabolism of fat helps the body eliminate accumulated body fat, which could precipitate the shedding of excess pounds. Additionally, adherents are also believed to experience a reduced appetite, which could lead to diminished caloric intake.

Keeping the weight off is important especially as adults age when they may need fewer calories daily compared to when living in there 20s or 30s even. Yet it is still important to get nutrient-rich food from this diet for older adults.

Protection Against Specific Illnesses

Keto dieters over age 50 could reduce their risk of developing ailments such as diabetes, mental disorders like Alzheimer's, various cardiovascular maladies, various kinds of cancer, Parkinson's Disease, Non-Alcoholic Fatty Liver Disease (NAFLD) and multiple sclerosis.

Aging

Aging is considered by some as the most important risk factor for human illnesses or disease. So reducing aging is the logical step to minimize these risk factors of disease.

Good news extending from the technical description of the ketosis process presented earlier shows the increased energy of youth as a result and because of the usage of fat as a fuel source, the body can go through a process where it can misinterpret signs so that the motor signal is suppressed and a lack of glucose is evident whereby it is reported aging may be slowed.

Generally, for years, multiple studies have noted that caloric restriction can aid in slowing aging and even increase lifespan. With the ketogenic diet, it is possible, without reducing calories to affect anti-aging. An intermittent fasting method used with the keto diet can also affect vascular aging.

Keto Dieting? Here Are 10 Foods You Must Have In Your Kitchen

The ketogenic diet is a very successful weight-loss program. It utilizes high fat and low carbohydrate ingredients to burn fat instead of glucose. Many people are familiar with the Atkins diet, but the keto plan restricts carbs even more. Because we are surrounded by fast-food restaurants and processed meals, it can be a challenge to avoid carb-rich foods, but proper planning can help.

Plan menus and snacks at least a week ahead of time, so you aren't caught with only high carb meal choices. Research keto recipes online; there are quite a few good ones to choose from. Immerse yourself in the keto lifestyle, find your favorite recipes, and stick with them.

There are a few items that are staples of a keto diet. Be sure to have these items on hand:

- Eggs - Used in omelets, quiches (yes, heavy cream is legal on keto!), hard-boiled as a snack, low carb pizza crust, and more; if you like eggs, you have a great chance of success on this diet
- Bacon - Do I need a reason? breakfast, salad garnish, burger topper, BLTs (no bread of course; try a BLT in a bowl, tossed in mayo)
- Cream cheese - Dozens of recipes, pizza crusts, main dishes, desserts
- Shredded cheese - Sprinkle over taco meat in a bowl, made into tortilla chips in the microwave, salad toppers, low-carb pizza and enchiladas
- Lots of romaine and spinach - Fill up on the green veggies; have plenty on hand for a quick salad when hunger pangs hit
- EZ-Sweetz liquid sweetener - Use a couple of drops in place of sugar; this artificial sweetener is the most natural and easiest to use that I've found
- Cauliflower - Fresh or frozen bags you can eat this low-carb veggie by itself, tossed in olive oil and baked, mashed in fake potatoes, chopped/shredded and used in place of rice under main dishes, in low-carb and keto pizza crusts, and much more
- Frozen chicken tenders - Have a large bag on hand; thaw quickly and grill, saute, mix with veggies and top with garlic sauce in a low carb flatbread, use in Chicken piccata, chicken alfredo, tacos, enchiladas, Indian Butter chicken, and more
- Ground beef - Make a big burger and top with all sorts of things from cheese, to sauteed mushrooms, to grilled onions... or crumble and cook with taco seasoning and use in provolone cheese taco shells; throw in a dish with lettuce, avocado, cheese, sour cream for a tortilla-less taco salad
- Almonds (plain or flavored) - these are a tasty and healthy snack; however, be sure to count them as you eat, because the

carbs DO add up. Flavors include habanero, coconut, salt and vinegar and more.

- The keto plan is a versatile and interesting way to lose weight, with lots of delicious food choices. Keep these 10 items stocked in your fridge, freezer, and larder, and you'll be ready to throw together some delicious keto meals and snacks at a moment's notice.

Side Effects of Using a Ketogenic Diet for Weight Loss

The ketogenic diet, colloquially called the keto diet, is a popular diet containing high amounts of fats, adequate-protein, and low carbohydrate. It is also referred to as a Low Carb-High Fat (LCHF) diet and a low carbohydrate diet. Ketogenic diets are designed to force the body to enter into a state called ketosis. The body generally makes use of carbohydrates as its primary source of energy. This owes to the fact that carbohydrates are the easiest for the body to absorb.

However, should the body run out of carbohydrates, it reverts to making use of fats and protein for its energy production. Ketosis effectively alters your body's natural equation from burning glucose to rather start burning fat as fuel. This alteration of the body's metabolism may come with some possible side effects as the body tries to adjust its functioning. Changing to the ketogenic diet is not that easy to adapt to especially at the initial onset. However, remember that these side effects are temporary. Some of them can last for a few days while others can last for months.

Therefore you need to give yourself time, both physically and mentally, to effectively make the switch. While making the switch to a ketogenic diet, there are two physical changes that you may experience. These are the keto flu and keto breath.

Keto Flu

This is one thing that anyone starting a ketogenic diet should brace up for. It is a condition in which you experience some of the different side effects that come along with using a ketogenic diet. Keto flu is often characterized by light-headedness or brain fogginess, headaches, nausea, stomachaches, and muscle soreness. You may also experience heightened feelings of lethargy, irritability and trouble concentrating.

Interestingly, these are all common symptoms of the flu, hence the name. These symptoms are temporary and not everyone using a ketogenic is affected by them. These symptoms are often caused by sugar withdrawal occasioned by the significantly reduced carbohydrate intake. Also, an imbalance in your body electrolytes such as calcium, magnesium, potassium, and sodium can affect how your body reacts to the effect of a ketogenic diet.

Keto Breath

There are two possible reasons put forth why people on ketogenic diets experience this peculiar breath issue. The body does not store ketones and thus they must be excreted from the body. Ketones can be excreted through the urine as acetoacetate. They can also be excreted through the breath in the form of acetone. So the more ketones you produce, the more acetone you pass out through your breath. Unfortunately, this can cause unpleasant-smelling breath when using a ketogenic diet.

On the other hand, increased protein ingestion can also cause keto breath. This is because the way the body digest fats and proteins is quite different. The digestion of proteins usually produces ammonia which the body excretes through the urine.

However, the increased consumption of proteins may result in the indigestible amounts remaining in your gut system and undergoes fermentation. This produces ammonia which is subsequently released through your breath. Keto breath can last for about a week to just under a month. It mostly depends on how well your body adapts to ketosis.

Micronutrient Deficiencies

This may result from the strict restrictions on carbohydrate intake. A lot of carbohydrate-rich foods are equally rich in vitamins and minerals. The severe restriction on carbohydrate intake may, therefore, cause deficiencies in some essential nutrients. Therefore, we should not only be focused on the micronutrient counting in terms of fat, proteins, and carbohydrates but should also remember the vitamin and mineral micronutrient contents as well.

This is often why supplements are mostly recommended when using a ketogenic diet. Supplementation will help to augment any micronutrient imbalance that might occur when using a ketogenic diet.

The Pros And Cons Of The Keto Diet

Let's talk about what ketosis is and what the science is saying about the diet. But first, let's cover the basics. The ketogenic diet is unique from other styles of eating because of its very high fat, and very low carbohydrate intake.

Ketogenesis may seem like a new concept, but it is the natural process your body reverts to when it does not have enough glucose to use as energy. Your body will begin to break down fat and create ketones as an energy source. It's kind of like your body's built-in backup generator!

Glucose is a form of sugar that is usually your body's (especially your brain's) main source of energy. When glucose is low, your body dips into your ketones that have been made from ketogenesis for energy. This alternative metabolic process your body switches to is known as ketosis. One job of your liver is to make ketones consistently anyway, but the amount will change based on one's carb and protein intake. The rate of generating ketones slows when it is simply not needed. But with the keto diet, your body doesn't get enough glucose to use it as its fuel. Instead, your body stays in a state of ketosis.

Possible Pros

- Epilepsy: The ketogenic diet was first used clinically to treat seizures. It has been used to successfully reduce seizures for many years, with research to back up the benefits outweighing any cons.
- Weight loss: There are some great metabolic changes initially with this diet. Notes that the health parameters associated with carrying excess weight improve, such as insulin resistance, high blood pressure, and elevated cholesterol and triglycerides. Fat oxidation does indeed increase due to the body adapting to the higher dietary fat intake.
- Type 2 diabetes: Carb restriction can have a direct impact on glucose concentrations, lowering them over time. It may be a straight forward way one could get their diabetes under control. But one should consult a registered dietitian before utilizing this strategy, as a general healthful diet and carb control can produce the same results.
- Cancer: This is a growing area of research for the ketogenic diet. The Warburg effect has established that tumor cells can break down glucose much faster (specifically 200x faster) compared to typical cells. The theory is that by "starving" tumor cells of glucose, you can inhibit their growth and help prevent cancer.

Possible Cons

Some negative side effects of a long-term ketogenic diet have been suggested in a review of the diet by Harvard's school of public health, including increased risk of kidney stones and osteoporosis, and increased blood levels of uric acid (a risk factor for gout). And the biggest areas of concern are shown below.

- Nutrient Deficiencies: Because whole food groups are excluded, nutrients typically found in foods like whole grains and fruit that are restricted from the diet can lead to deficiencies, especially if the diet is followed incorrectly or without proper guidance. It is vital to incorporate a wide variety of foods while eating such high amounts of fat. Each food group offers different essential nutrition. Focus on meats, seafood, vegetables, some legumes, and fruits to make sure you are getting fiber, B vitamins, and minerals such as iron, magnesium, and zinc. It would be best to consult with a registered dietitian to alleviate the possibility of any deficiencies.

- Keto Flu: During the diet transition you may experience uncomfortable side effects from significantly cutting carbs, sometimes called the "Keto Flu". Hunger, headaches, nausea, fatigue, irritability, constipation and brain "fog" may last days. Sleep and hydration will help, but it may not be a pleasant transition into the diet.

- Adherence: Point blank, following a very high-fat diet, may be challenging to maintain for most. Keeping yourself satisfied with a limited variety of food and food groups and not being allowed to have some of the more pleasurable foods like fruit, rice dishes, ice cream, or cream-based soups may be challenging to maintain. This is very individual, but adhering to a healthy diet is important. To truly gain long-term health benefits, one must have healthy habits in place year-round, not 30 days at a time.

- Gut Health: Using the restroom may be difficult since removing whole grain and fruit will greatly lower one's fiber intake. Not great for gut health.

Dos And Don'ts Of The Keto Diet

If you're ready to try following the ketogenic diet, then you need to set yourself up for success from day one. Below are some dos and don'ts to keep in mind when you first begin.

Dos:

- Stick with healthy fats like eggs, avocado, and extra virgin olive oil
- Eat low-carb greens as much as possible to maximize your nutrient intake
- Eat real food made from whole ingredients (nothing processed)
- Source organic, grass-fed animal products as much as possible
- Stay hydrated- it helps offset the loss of fiber in your diet
- Keep a food journal to track how you feel over time
- Consider a modified keto diet if the restrictions are too severe
- Consult with your doctor before beginning if you have underlying medical conditions
- Consider nutritional coaching to ensure you follow the eating plan correctly
- Replace your electrolytes by drinking bone broth

Don'ts:

- Avoid eating fast food as much as possible (the fat content is low quality, even in keto-friendly meals)
- Don't avoid looking at nutritional information before you eat- most foods have more carbs than you would expect
- Avoid "bad fats" like corn, soybean, canola or hydrogenated oil
- Avoid any processed food listed as low-fat, as most manufacturers make up for the lack of flavor with extra sugar (carbs)
- Don't overeat. The high satiety of keto-friendly food might mean that your place looks emptier at mealtimes than it did before. Avoid overstuffing yourself out of habit.
- Don't stress about calories. There's little reason to monitor your amounts if your macronutrient ratios are where they should be.
- Avoid consuming too many nuts or dairy products, as they are typically calorie-dense and are easy to overeat.

Frequently Asked Questions

Here are answers to some of the most common questions about the ketogenic diet.

1. Can I Ever Eat Carbs Again?

Yes. However, it is important to significantly reduce your carb intake initially. After the first 2–3 months, you can eat carbs on special occasions just return to the diet immediately after.

2. Will I Lose Muscle?

There is a risk of losing some muscle on any diet. However, the high protein intake and high ketone levels may help minimize muscle loss, especially if you lift weights.

3. Can I Build Muscle On A Ketogenic Diet?

Yes, but it may not work as well as on a moderate-carb diet.

4. Do I Need To Refeed Or Carb Load?

No. However, a few higher-calorie days may be beneficial now and then.

5. How Much Protein Can I Eat?

Protein should be moderate, as a very high intake can spike insulin levels and lower ketones. Around 35% of the total calorie intake is probably the upper limit.

6. What If I Am Constantly Tired, Weak Or Fatigued?

You may not be in full ketosis or be utilizing fats and ketones efficiently. To counter this, lower your carb intake and re-visit the points above. A supplement like MCT oil or ketones may also help.

7. My Urine Smells Fruity. Why Is This?

Don't be alarmed. This is simply due to the excretion of by-products created during ketosis.

8. My Breath Smells. What Can I Do?

This is a common side effect. Try drinking naturally flavored water or chewing sugar-free gum.

9. I Heard Ketosis Was Extremely Dangerous. Is This True?

People often confuse ketosis with ketoacidosis. The former is natural, while the latter only occurs in uncontrolled diabetes. Ketoacidosis is dangerous, but the ketosis on a ketogenic diet is perfectly normal and healthy.

10. I Have Digestion Issues And Diarrhea. What Can I Do?

This common side effect usually passes after 3–4 weeks. If it persists, try eating more high-fiber veggies. Magnesium supplements can also help with constipation.

CHAPTER 6 : SCIENTIFIC FACTS ABOUT INTERMITTENT FASTING

The Science Behind Intermittent Fasting

"One of the major keys to understanding fasting, to understanding any diet, is understanding the role insulin plays," Dr. Hutchins says. Insulin, the hormone that regulates blood sugar, is made in the pancreas and released in the bloodstream in response to eating. Once released, insulin causes the body to store energy as fat. "Insulin makes fat, so the more insulin made, the more fat you store," he says.

During intermittent fasting, the periods when you are not eating give the body time to lower insulin levels, which reverses the fat-storing process. "When insulin levels drop, the process goes in reverse and you lose fat. With more leptin and less ghrelin, people will feel fuller faster and hungry less often, which could translate to fewer calories consumed and, as a result, weight loss.

Health Benefits of Intermittent Fasting

Besides losing weight, people who fast may experience improved heart and brain functions because of reduced insulin.

"Think of your insulin level as the first domino in the whole-body cascade of what can happen with intermittent fasting," Dr. Hutchins says. "If you have high insulin levels, that can lead to obesity, diabetes, high blood pressure, and elevated triglycerides. Those things together are called metabolic syndrome, which increases the risk of cardiovascular disease. So, if your insulin level decreases, you will probably lose weight, and your cholesterol, blood sugar and blood pressure will improve.”

The drop in cholesterol can also decrease the inflammation caused by metabolic syndrome, namely plaque buildup in the arteries and overall cardiovascular inflammation. “As a result of these improvements, people can also reduce their risk of cardiovascular disease,” he adds.

This process can happen even in the absence of weight loss, and Dr. Hutchins notes that it’s not specific to intermittent fasting. “Some people can intermittently fast and be on a strict regimen, but if they eat a bunch of junk on the days they can eat, the diet won’t affect heart health,” he says. “This effect is probably more specific to what they’re eating than to when they’re eating.”

When it comes to the brain, Dr. Hutchins says that some data has shown that lower insulin levels can also reduce dysfunction in a person’s brain cells, called neurons, which could decrease the risk of Parkinson’s and Alzheimer’s diseases. “But this is still only theoretical. Risk of Alzheimer’s, for example, is significantly higher in people who have metabolic syndrome.”

Should You Try Intermittent Fasting?

Although intermittent fasting might bring health benefits, Dr. Hutchins emphasizes that whether you see results in weight loss or overall health comes down to nutrition.

“Based on the data I have looked at, I can’t say that intermittent fasting is more successful than other diets that aren’t on a fasting pattern,” he says. “The problem I have found with intermittent fasting is that people can stick with the fasting, but when they start a period where they are eating again, they end up eating a lot of junk and processed food instead of healthy food.”

Ultimately, Dr. Hutchins says the best diet is the one that works best for you. He says there’s no perfect candidate for intermittent fasting, but if you want to try the diet, find a fasting schedule that fits in with your lifestyle. For example, if fasting one full day is too hard, try eating for eight hours and fasting for 16 instead.

Always, the main emphasis of your diet should be on what you're eating. "The bottom line is you have to be eating real food, not processed stuff," Dr. Hutchins says. "I'd recommend eating a lower-carbohydrate diet, limiting both sweets and starches, because those are the things that cause your insulin level to rise most."

It's also important during periods of fasting that you remain hydrated. "When people fast, they aren't fasting from water," he says. "You have to stay well-hydrated."

Like any other diet, people should also consider medications when altering their eating habits. For example, people on blood pressure medicine or medication that lowers their blood sugar should avoid fasting, as periods of not eating could cause blood sugar levels to drop too low, resulting in hypoglycemia, a serious complication of low blood sugar levels. Talk to your doctor about the diet that is best for you, and before you pursue any kind of fasting.

Is Intermittent Fasting Safe And Healthy?

Yes, intermittent fasting does have a lot of benefits. We talk about them in our 21-Day Intermittent Fasting Challenge a lot. It is also a good time to say that this article should and does not intend to replace advice from your doctor and you should always consult your physician before planning any fasting and especially extended fasting (longer than 24h). Now that we made it clear, here are some of the cases (but might not be limited to) that does not go well with intermittent fasting:

- If you have a diabetes
- If you take medications for blood pressure or heart disease
- If you are pregnant or breastfeeding
- If you have a history of disordered eating
- If you don't sleep well

- If you are under 18 years old

Also, you should be a lot more careful if you are practicing extended fasting, which depending on the source you follow will be continuous fasting for either anything more than 24, 48 or 72 hours. There is a consensus that any fasts longer than 72 hours should be done under strict medical supervision.

What Is Fasting?

The way we as scientists who study fasting define it is not consuming food for a long enough period to elevate the levels of compounds called ketones. In the fed state that is, when you're not fasting glucose is the primary fuel used by cells, including neurons. Fasting depletes the liver's store of glucose, prompting fat cells to release fats. The fats travel to the liver where they're converted into ketones, which are essentially small pieces of fats that cells can use as an energy source.

This metabolic switch going from using glucose to using ketones as an energy source happens after about 10 to 14 hours of not consuming food, depending on how active you are. Exercise will accelerate the onset of the switch.

There are different types of fasting regimens. In lab animals, the main regimen we use is alternate-day fasting where the rats or mice have no food for 24 hours, followed by a 24-hour period where they can eat, and so on. Alternatively, you can restrict the number of time animals has access to food to a four- to the six-hour window so that they're fasting between 18 and 20 hours a day. In people, we've studied a fasting regimen called the 5:2 diet, where people eat normally for five days out of the week and then eat only about 500 calories on the other two days.

Intermittent Fasting Impacts Brain Function

Fasting has phenomenal advantages over a range of different brain functions. Perhaps the most significant of these comes from a cellular cleansing process known as autophagy activation. Humans and mammals alike respond in similar ways when they are deprived severely from calories, and the size of most of their major organs will shrink, that is, except for the brain and the testicles. It is said that this is to protect the survival of these species and it makes a lot of sense, on both counts.

What is Autophagy Activation?

Autophagy is essentially where the body will eat itself. It sounds a little scary, but it is one of the best things you can train your body to do. It is the natural way for the body to clean itself from the inside out.

Autophagy plays a crucial role in your body's ability to regenerate, repair and detoxifies itself. By activating this process, you can reduce inflammation, optimize your brain functions and slow down the aging process. Plenty of research has been conducted which proves that fasting promotes autophagy within the brain. It can increase neuroplasticity, cognitive functions and improve brain structure. Intermittent fasting is a proven way to activate autophagy.

Recent Studies Showing The Effects Of Fasting On Brain Function

Professor Mark Mattson, the current Chief of the Laboratory of Neuroscience at the National Institute on Ageing and Professor of Neuroscience at The Johns Hopkins University, gave a TEDx talk on the subject of fasting and its effects on the brain. He reported studies showed fasting caused positive neurochemical changes to occur in the brains of test subjects, which lead to an improvement of cognitive function and resistance to stressful stimuli. These studies also showed calorific restriction reduced inflammation in the brain and increased neurotrophic factors such as the production and growth of neurons (which help with learning and memory).

Professor Mattson also reported studies indicated fasting constitutes a challenge to the brain. The brain reacts to this challenge by adapting response pathways to help it cope with stress.

Interestingly, Professor Mattson outlined the brain's reaction to intermittent fasting is the same reaction it has to regular exercise. Both activities affect increasing protein production in the brain, which then promotes the growth and connection of neurons and strengthens synapses. Both practices also stimulate the production of nerve cells in the hippocampus, stimulates the production of ketones ("petrol" for neurons) and increases the number of mitochondria within neurons, which in turn help the neurons to maintain their connections. All of this has the net effect of improving memory and increasing the ability to learn.

He also said there were some indications "intermittent fasting enhances the ability of nerve cells to repair DNA." If this is the case, it may be a good topic for research to concentrate on when examining preventative measures and possible treatment conditions such as Dystonia and Dementia. In fact, according to Professor Mattson, some research that has been in this space has already shown positive results.

One aspect of the research particularly interesting to note is that benefits were not related to a calorific restriction in general, but with specific intentional periods of intermittent fasting.

All indications show that intermittent fasting not only has positive effects on your body, like weight loss and improvement of risk factors in respect of heart disease, diabetes and the like; it also has an extremely positive effect on your brain, allowing increased levels of focus and memory retention.

Intermittent fasting, in particular, may lead to improvements in memory and learning, as well as developing a greater resistance in the brain to conditions such as Dystonia, and Dementia.

What Is BDNF?

Think of brain-derived neurotrophic factors as fertilizer for your brain. You have billions of neurons (aka brain cells), and BDNF keeps them flourishing and strong. When you release BDNF, it flips the switch on a series of genes that grow brand-new brain cells and pathways. BDNF also strengthens the neurons you already have. Along with keeping you mentally alert and improving memory, high BDNF carries loads of other benefits, too.

Benefits Of High BDNF

Increases Brain Plasticity

When your brain cells get damaged or face a stressful situation, BDNF protects them and helps them come back stronger.

Eases Depression

Your neural pathways become more flexible instead of shutting down, which could explain why higher levels of a brain-derived neurotrophic factor are associated with warding off depression.

Boosts Weight Loss

BDNF can help you lose weight. Studies show that the more overweight a person is, the lower their BDNF levels. One study suggests that, at least in mice, lowering levels of BDNF did make them more prone to obesity.

Improves Sleep

Brain-derived neurotrophic factor can help you sleep better by increasing your slow brain waves during your deepest stage of sleep.

How To Increase BDNF

1. Exercise

Endurance exercise releases a protein called FNDC5 (fibronectin type III domain-containing protein 5. How's that for a mouthful?). FNDC5, in turn, increases brain-derived neurotrophic factor by 200-300 percent. In another study, men who cycled daily for 3 months nearly quadrupled their resting BDNF.

Strength training increases BDNF, but only for a few minutes post-workout. Opt for moderately intense cardio, as Mark Sisson recommends in this Bulletproof Radio podcast episode. Not a fan of running? Swim, cycle, do fast-paced yoga or pick up a sport. Whatever gets your heart rate going will increase BDNF levels as well.

2. Deep Sleep

You release a brain-derived neurotrophic factor during the deeper stages of sleep. There are four sleep stages, and you cycle through them every 90 minutes or so. On average, you spend about a third to half the night in stages 3 and 4, the ones that give you deep, restorative sleep.

With a few hacks, though, you can drop into deep sleep faster and stay there longer in each sleep cycle. That means more BDNF release and better rest in less time. Learn how to sleep better with these sleep hacks.

3. Meditation

Stress is toxic to BDNF. No surprise, then, that meditation increases BDNF, specifically strengthening areas of the brain that correlate with pain tolerance, body awareness, meta-thinking (awareness of how you think), memory, emotional control, happiness, and attention.

Start by meditating for 5 minutes every morning. Some days you may quiet your mind, while other days your thoughts may run rampant. When beginning a meditation practice, don't get too attached to the results. Consistency is more important than "getting it right." Make it a habit with this 30-day meditation challenge for beginners.

4. Psychedelics

Both psilocybin (mushrooms) and LSD (acid) increase BDNF production and neurogenesis. That could explain why there are so many studies coming out about psychedelic-assisted therapy helping with depression and PTSD — perhaps the combination allows people to rapidly rewire the stubborn pathways that are causing them pain.

Here's a breakdown of several psychedelics. These psychedelics are probably illegal where you live, and they can cause psychological distress if you take them without care. Remember to always responsibly.

5. Polyphenols

These antioxidants stimulate brain-derived neurotrophic factor and protect your brain from stress. Coffee, green tea, dark chocolate, blueberries, and colorful vegetables are all excellent polyphenol sources.

Coffee fruit extract (the red fruit surrounding coffee beans) is especially potent, and 100 mg of coffee fruit extract raised BDNF by about 140 percent in several studies. The boost lasted for a few hours. The coffee fruit extract is a useful supplement to add to your brain hacking toolbox.

6. Hypoxia

Depriving your brain of oxygen for a brief period triggers instant BDNF release. You can do this any time in under two minutes with simple breathing exercises like the Wim Hof method.

7. Sunlight

Simple sun exposure increases brain-derived neurotrophic factor. It also improves mood, increases vitamin D production, and decreases your risk of skin cancer, provided you don't burn yourself. Get outside in direct sunlight for 10-20 minutes a day. Leave your sunscreen and sunglasses at home. You want the UV rays hitting photoreceptors on your skin and in your retinas.

8. Intermittent Fasting

Intermittent fasting when you eat all your daily calories during a set period increases your BDNF. In one study, mice with Huntington's disease — a neurodegenerative disorder who were put on an intermittent fasting diet showed a slower progression of the disease than mice fed a normal diet. The fasting mice had higher levels of BDNF, suggesting that intermittent fasting can boost the production of this protein, and therefore protect against brain atrophy.

What Blocks BDNF?

Stress: Stress is one of the biggest BDNF inhibitors. You're constantly bombarded with work, advertisements, information, pollution, artificial lighting, and all kinds of other stimuli that tax your biology. Make it a part of your day to manage your stress.

Sugar. Eating sugar, and fructose in particular directly curbs BDNF production in rats and links to cognitive decline in humans. That doesn't mean you have to cut out sweets, though. Swap sugar for one of these high-quality alternative sweeteners (not Splenda or aspartame). And if you're struggling with sugar cravings, try taking this 30-day no sugar challenge.

6 Surprising Brain Power Benefits of Intermittent Fasting

Intermittent fasting is not a new concept fasting has been utilized for health and longevity for centuries. The health benefits of fasting are numerous and extensive, especially as more research has validated the benefits of intermittent fasting for not only weight loss but many other aspects of our health.

1. Reduces Inflammation

Intermittent fasting has been shown to significantly reduce inflammation. Excessive inflammation is the cause of many chronic diseases that we face today including Alzheimer's, dementia, obesity diabetes, and more. There are many methods that show how intermittent fasting reduces inflammation.

• Autophagy: Autophagy is when the body destroys old or damaged cells. Think of it like cleaning off the rust and cleansing itself. It's a way of the body repairing itself. If old or damaged cells remain in the body, they create inflammation. Intermittent fasting stimulates autophagy, helping the body to cleanse itself, thereby reducing inflammation

• Ketones: During fasting, the body uses up all of its sugar stores and has to turn to fat for fuel. When fats get broken down it creates ketones. One of the most abundant ketones, β-hydroxybutyrate, actually blocks part of the immune system responsible for regulating inflammatory disorders like arthritis and even Alzheimer's.

• Insulin Sensitivity: Fasting has been shown to help resolve insulin resistance. When the body becomes resistant to insulin, insulin and glucose build up in the blood and create inflammation. Intermittent fasting allows your body to take a break. Since there is no food to digest and your body uses up all it's sugar stores, insulin levels begin to drop, allowing the body to re-sensitize to insulin again.

2. Create More Brain Cells

Seriously! You can create more brain cells and therefore improve your brain power. According to Dr. Mark Mattson, a professor of Neurology at John Hopkins University, fasting has been shown to increase rates of neurogenesis in the brain. Neurogenesis is the growth and development of new brain cells and nerve tissues. Higher rates of neurogenesis are linked to increasing brain performance, memory, mood, and focus. One particular study showed that intermittent fasting (the researchers used a 16:8 schedule in the study) stimulated the production of new brain cells.

3. Boost "Miracle Grow" In Your Brain

Not only does fasting increase your rate of neurogenesis, but it also boosts the production of an important protein called BDNF. BDNF has been hailed as "Miracle Grow For Your Brain."

BDNF has been shown to play a role in neuroplasticity, which allows the brain to continue to change and adapt. It makes your brain more resilient to stress and more adaptable to change. BDNF helps to produce new brain cells, protect your brain cells, stimulate new connections and synapses while also boosting memory, improving mood, and learning. Intermittent fasting has been shown to boost BDNF by 50–400%!

4. Burns Fat for Fuel Instead Of Sugar

This may come as a shock, but fat is a better and cleaner source of fuel than carbohydrates. Not only does fat produce more energy per gram than carbohydrates do, but it produces less free radicals, which cause inflammation. When your mitochondria, your cells batteries, use fat (ketones) or carbohydrates to make energy, there is waste that gets produces in the form of free radicals.

Free radicals cause oxidative stress to the body and are thought to be the cause of many chronic diseases we face today, including many neurodegenerative diseases. Intermittent fasting forces your brain to use ketones, rather than sugar, which is cleaner and more efficient fuel for your brain.

5. Boosts Human Growth Hormone

Upon first hearing human growth hormone (HGH), you may have a picture of a bodybuilder using it to get huge muscles. HGH from an exogenous source (from the outside) is not recommended for a wide variety of reasons and isn't the best for your body. HGH has been discovered to have incredibly powerful anti-aging and longevity benefits, but in particular, HGH can improve cognition, provide neuroprotection, and increase neurogenesis.

One study, in particular, showed that HGH had a neuroprotective effect, preserving your brain health and brain performance. Intermittent fasting has been shown to naturally boost HGH levels to provide healthy anti-aging, repair, neuroprotective, and longevity benefits.

6. Supercharges Your Energy

Intermittent Fasting has been shown to boost mitochondrial biogenesis, the creation of new mitochondria. As we've mentioned earlier, mitochondria are the batteries power your cells to do their job. Their job is to take the food you eat and turn it into energy. Mitochondria in the brain help your brain have more brainpower.

Fasting

fasting as to abstain from food or to eat sparingly or abstain from some foods. Fasting done correctly is the total elimination of food for several hours or days. Only water is taken in the body, which allows the body to restore itself to optimal health.

You may hear people refer to "juice" fasts, where the only food taken in is fruit and vegetable juices but that is not a true fast. The "Juice Fasts" should be called juice feasts as most proponents of juicing will take in nearly the same amount of calories as they would whole food during their regular nutrition schedule. No food is eaten during a true fast.

There are a significant number of people that practice "Natural Hygiene" where one of the major components is fasting done to cleanse the system of toxins and restore the body to health. Most fasting proponents will fast for short periods at least 2 times annually.

During the fast other therapies may also be used which help aid in the elimination of waste from your body. The use of exercise, colonics, sunlight, meditation, yoga stretching, tai chi, and Pilates as well as making sure the body gets plenty of rest are ways to assist the detoxification process.

Fasting has been reported to be effective in treating high blood pressure, headaches, allergies, arthritis, and other inflammatory conditions, psychological problems, obesity, high cholesterol, lethargy, and general malaise. Fasting done properly is a low cost and effective therapy for a wide range of health-related problems. Long fasts should only be undertaken with the aid of an experienced fasting supervisor.

Fasting should always be pursued gradually and you should be particularly cautious when breaking a fast. For example, when I conduct a seven-day juice fast, it requires 10 to 12 days to complete the entire cleansing program. I pre-fast on fresh fruits for at least 2 days, followed by 7 days on freshly squeezed fruit juices and water, followed by at least 2 days on fresh fruits. After that, I incrementally introduce raw vegetables and cooked vegetables to my diet until my stomach regains full digestive power. During the fasting period, it may be necessary to employ water enemas to assist the elimination of wastes in the intestines.

Break fasts by eating very slowly, chewing very thoroughly and eating very small portions. I find 7 days on juice is relatively easy, but breaking the fast for the next several days is quite hard for me to handle because it requires even greater self-control. Throughout my fasting period, I always give myself at least a full hour of Reiki self-healing each day.

Leptin A Hormone That Regulates Body Weight

Leptin is a hormone that is produced by your body's fat cells, It is often referred to as the "satiety hormone" or the "starvation hormone." Leptin's primary target is in the brain particularly an area called the hypothalamus. Leptin is supposed to tell your brain that when you have enough fat stored you don't need to eat and can burn calories at a normal rate. It also has many other functions related to fertility, immunity and brain function.

However, leptin's main role is long-term regulation of energy, including the number of calories you eat and expend, as well as how much fat you store in your body. The leptin system evolved to keep humans from starving or overeating, both of which would have made you less likely to survive in the natural environment. Today, leptin is very effective at keeping us from starving. But something is broken in the mechanism that is supposed to prevent us from overeating.

What Is Leptin Resistance?

People who are obese have a lot of body fat in their fat cells. Because fat cells produce leptin in proportion to their size, people who are obese also have very high levels of leptin. Given the way leptin is supposed to work, many obese people should naturally limit their food intake. In other words, their brains should know that they have plenty of energy stored. However, their leptin signaling may not work. While copious leptin may be present, the brain doesn't see it.

This condition known as leptin resistance is now believed to be one of the main biological contributors to obesity. When your brain doesn't receive the leptin signal, it erroneously thinks that your body is starving even though it has more than enough energy stored.

This makes your brain change its behavior to regain body fat. Your brain then encourages:

- Eating More: Your brain thinks that you must eat to prevent starvation.
- Reduced Energy Expenditure: To conserve energy, your brain decreases your energy levels and makes you burn fewer calories at rest.

Thus, eating more and exercising less is not the underlying cause of weight gain but rather a possible consequence of leptin resistance, a hormonal defect. For most people who struggle with leptin resistance, willing yourself to overcome the leptin-driven starvation signal is next to impossible.

Impact On Dieting

Leptin resistance may be one reason that many diets fail to promote long-term weight loss. If you're leptin-resistant, losing weight still reduces fat mass, which leads to a significant reduction in leptin levels

— but your brain doesn't necessarily reverse its leptin resistance. When leptin goes down, this leads to hunger, increased appetite, reduced motivation to exercise and a decreased number of calories burned at rest.

Your brain then thinks that you are starving and initiates various powerful mechanisms to regain that lost body fat. This could be the main reason why so many people yo-yo diet and lose a significant amount of weight only to gain it back shortly thereafter.

What Causes Leptin Resistance?

Several potential mechanisms behind leptin resistance have been identified.

These include:

- Inflammation: Inflammatory signaling in your hypothalamus is likely an important cause of leptin resistance in both animals and humans.
- Free Fatty Acids: Having elevated free fatty acids in your bloodstream may increase fat metabolites in your brain and interfere with leptin signaling.
- Having High Leptin: Having elevated levels of leptin in the first place seems to cause leptin resistance.

Most of these factors are amplified by obesity, meaning that you could get trapped in a vicious cycle of gaining weight and becoming increasingly leptin resistant over time.

Can Leptin Resistance Be Reversed?

Focusing on an overall healthy lifestyle is also likely to be an effective strategy.

There are several things you can do:

- Avoid Processed Food: Highly processed foods may compromise the integrity of your gut and drive inflammation.
- Eat Soluble Fiber: Eating soluble fiber can help improve your gut health and may protect against obesity.
- Exercise: Physical activity may help reverse leptin resistance
- Sleep: Poor sleep is implicated in problems with leptin. Lower your triglycerides: Having high triglycerides can prevent the transport of leptin from your blood to your brain. The best way to lower triglycerides is to reduce your carb intake.
- Eat Protein: Eating plenty of protein can cause automatic weight loss, which may result from an improvement in leptin sensitivity.

Though there is no simple way to eliminate leptin resistance, you can make long-term lifestyle changes that may improve your quality of life.

Here you seem to have another question: If it is all the matter of hormone and brain processes, can we do anything to influence it? Well, we can, at least to some extent.

We can deceive our body and not eat more than necessary. And lose weight this way. Here are some tips:

- Don't go hungry! Have a bite during the day;
- Never omit a meal in the morning. It will help you not to be so much hungry in the evening;
- Eat slowly, don't hasten;
- Don't put all the dishes on the table. The more you have to wait until you continue eating, the better;
- If it is possible, make a pause during the meal. Wait for the moment when you suddenly realize you are not hungry anymore.

All these tips will let the leptin level increase and the appetite will be inhibited. You will stop eating and gaining excess body weight. Gradually, day after day, you will even begin to lose it.

7 Fast And Fun Fat Burning Facts

Here are seven fast and fun facts for effectively burning fat:

1. Drink a glass of milk immediately upon rising in the morning. A tall glass of nonfat or 2% milk will help you break your fast from the night before. The protein will give you energy and help to remove any hunger pangs.

2. Take a supplement rich in zinc to help you keep the pounds off. Just an increase in zinc makes leptin levels rise; which causes your body to build muscle instead of fat. Leptin is a hormone that helps regulate body fat by telling your body when you're satisfied.

3. Burn approximately eight 1/2 pounds a year just by doing two minutes of push-ups every morning as soon as you get out of bed.

4. Avoid becoming weight obsessive when you begin your fat burning program. Instead of simply shooting for weight reduction, focus on what that result will do for another part of your life.

5. To cut your pounds down to size de-stress your life. Stress releases cortisol into your bloodstream. This hormone also affects your body fat level adversely. Learning how to handle stress effectively will reduce your levels of cortisol and help you to strip the fat.

6. Walk it off for better health. A half-hour walks a day positively influences your mood. The simple act of taking a walk can help you de-stress while increasing your activity level.

7. A jump rope is the perfect fat burning tool. 10 minutes of continuous exercise with a jump rope is equal to 30 minutes of jogging.

CHAPTER 7: COMMON MISTAKES TO AVOID

Most people face difficulty in carrying on with the process of intermittent fasting because their approach to the whole process is completely wrong. Being actively aware of the proper methods while deciding on undertaking intermittent fasting might turn out to be the main difference between failure and success. Here are some of the most common mistakes that people make while undergoing the process of intermittent fasting that needs to be avoided for getting the ultimate re- sults.

Using The Method As A Reason For Eating Rubbish

Well, many people think of the process of intermittent fasting just like a magic pill that can solve all the problems that they are having. It is true that intermittent fast- ing is actually a great tool for taking complete control over your health. But it won't be able to completely cancel out your habit of having processed foods all the time. At the time of intermittent fasting, you are required to nourish the body with all types of nutrient-rich and whole food items. When your body is in the state of fast- ing, your body will start breaking down all the components that are damaged in na- ture and will use them up for providing energy. This whole process will clean up and heal your body. This also means that your body will tend to become more sensitive to the types of food that you are going to eat. It will be great if you are having food items that are rich in nutrients and not having anything that is rubbish. Also, when you fail to nourish the body with foods that are dense in nutrients, you will go through extreme feelings of hunger as your body will be craving for nutrients. So, using this process as the key to eat rubbish is not going to help you in any way.

Restricting Calories During The Eating Phase

The primary issue that most of the people face as they start with the process of intermittent fasting is that they try to restrict their calorie intake as they break their fast. The overall point of following intermittent fasting is to properly listen to the body and continue eating until you are full. The human body is a great machine only if you permit it to do its job in the proper way. Our body releases hormones for making us feel full when it understands that it does not need any more food. When you try to restrict your calorie intake at the time of eating, you might end up eating much less than you actually need. This will ultimately result in causing var- ious unwanted changes in your body that might not be a really good thing for you.

Trying To Do Several Things All At Once – Under Eat, Fast, and Over Train

There is a very popular saying, 'Do not try to bite off more if you cannot chew.' If you have several years by eating in a bad way and without exercising and you want to opt for intermittent fasting, it is better not to overdo things. Try to ease yourself up with the process of fasting and start training gradually. Do not just start with training five times a week, every day fasting and calorie restriction as you eat from the first day. This overall combination might result in various types of serious problems. Your body needs a little amount of physical stress but stressing too much might result in chronic issues.

Getting Obsessed With Eating Windows And Timings

One of the primary benefits of intermittent fasting is that it can teach you to under- stand your body. You will learn to understand what is meant by real hunger of the body which is something that generally occurs after every 18-24 hours and not after every 3-4 hours. Your body will be dictating when you need to eat and not the

ticking clock. If you try to focus only on the time periods, you will only end up counting down the total hours until which you can consume food. You are never going to learn how to understand the signals of your body.

Not Having Enough Water

When your body enters the state of fasting, it begins to break down all the dam- aged components and thus detoxifies your body. It is of utter importance that you throw all of these toxins out of your body by drinking enough water. As you start fasting, try to have as much water as you can have. Also, drinking water throughout your period of fasting can help in making you feel full which is really important as you start with intermittent fasting.

Allowing Fasting To Rule Over Your Life

We all love the company of our family and friends. But, as you start with the process of intermittent fasting, you might get inclined to cancel dinner with friends or any party only because you are fasting. In this way, it might turn out to be not so enjoyable for the long term. Do not allow the fasting periods to rule over your life. Try shifting your routine backward or forward only by a few hours on those days when you have got some sort of plans with your family or friends. Intermittent fast- ing is much more than a program; it is a lifestyle that needs to be properly mingled with your regular life. It is flexible in nature and so there is no meaning of canceling all your social plans. Just alter your routine a bit and you are good to go.

Overeating During The Eating Phase

It is very easy to overeat right after you are done with your fasting period as you might feel hungry or just want to justify yourself that you are actually filling up the calories that have been lost. This whole thinking might backfire if you are

practicing intermittent fasting for losing weight. So, try to prepare some healthy meals as your fast ends and try to keep as many whole food items as possible in the diet. Do not overeat than you usually do and try keeping it normal.

CHAPTER 8: EXERCISES TO LOSE WEIGHT

Carrying around excessive weight always feels uncomfortable and moreover it can impact your overall health. The rates of obesity have reached new heights in the past few years. Obesity can be regarded as the storehouse of all types of diseases and thus can lead to numerous chronic health-related problems. The most com- mon problems that arise from obesity are diabetes, heart diseases, several types of cancer, stroke, and others. A person can lose excess body weight by limiting the total calorie intake via their diet. The second way of dealing with it is by burning down extra calories with the help of exercise.

Benefits of Exercise

The most effective way of losing weight is by combining your regular healthy diet with exercise in place of just focusing on calorie restriction. Exercise comes with the power of preventing and even reversing the effects of various diseases. As you start with exercising, you can easily lower the level of cholesterol along with blood pressure of your body which can help in preventing the chances of a heart attack. Exercise can also prevent the development of various types of cancers like breast cancer and colon cancer. It can also provide you with a sense of well-being along with confidence. Thus, it can lower the rates of depression and anxiety. Exercise is also very helpful for losing weight and also for maintaining the loss of weight. It can help in improving your body's metabolism. With daily exercising, you can also increase and maintain your lead muscle mass which directly helps in in- creasing the total number of calories that you can burn in a day.

How Much Exercise Is Required For Losing Weight?

For reaping all the health-related benefits of exercising, it is always suggested that

you engage yourself in some sort of aerobic exercise for a minimum session of 20 minutes for at least 3 times every week. But, if possible by you, you can easily ex- tend the session more than 20 minutes that will actually help you in losing weight. When you include only 10-15 minutes of very moderate exercise, for example, walk- ing or jogging for a mile, on a regular basis, it can help you in burning almost 100 extra calories. As you burn around 700 calories every week, it can equate to almost 10 lbs. of weight loss all throughout the course of the year.

Including Exercise Into Your Daily Routine

The amount of exercise that you can actually incorporate in your daily life values more than you perform it in one session. That is the reason why bringing about small changes in your regular routine can bring about a big difference in the size of your waistline. You can consider several healthy habits that you can include in your lifestyle such as:

•Riding your cycle or walking to your workplace.

•Omitting the elevator and taking the stairs.

•Parking your car at far away distances and walk along the distance in between.

Is It Possible To Exercise While Fasting?

If you are practicing intermittent fasting for losing weight or for any other reasons and you are willing to get along with your workout routine, there are certain pros and cons that you need to consider. Some research depicted that if you exercise at the time of fasting, it can affect the biochemistry of your muscles. It might also af- fect the body's metabolism that is directly linked to a steady level of blood sugar and sensitivity to insulin. Some research suggests that exercising while fasting helps in depleting the stored form of carbohydrates, also known as glycogen, and thus you will be burning more amount of stored fat. Also, exercising with an empty stomach helps in speeding up the fat-burning process. So, it can be said that exercising while fasting comes with mixed type of support, where some say that it is good for health while some say it is not.

Thinking About The Timing

For making your workout session more effective in nature at the time of fasting, you are required to think about the time which is ideal for you. You need to find out whether you should opt for working out during, before, or right after the window of eating. Working out right before the eating window is ideal for those people who perform their best at the time of working out on an empty stomach. People who cannot perform their exercise with an empty stomach can opt for exercising during the eating window. Such people can effectively capitalize on the nutrition of post- workout. And, if you think you can get the best out of yourself right after fueling, you can opt for exercising after having your meal. No matter the time that you choose, try to decide it only after listening to the responses of the body. You can experiment with the various time slots and find out when your body performs the best.

How To Carry On With Safe Exercising At The Time Of Fasting

The success rate of any program of exercise or weight loss depends completely on the extent of how safe it is for sustaining over the long run. If your aim is to reduce your body fat percentage and also maintain your level of fitness while performing intermittent fasting, you are required to be in the safe zone. Let's have a look at some of the tips.

Having a meal close to your workout session: The timing of yo ur meal can play a very big role in your workout session. The key to reaping all the benefits of a work- out session is to time your meal close to the workout session. This way your body can easily tap in the stored glycogen in the body for fueling your session of work- out. Also, you can include some protein supplements right after working out for gaining more lean muscles.

•**Staying hydrated:** Fasting does not mean that you cannot have wat er. Drink-

ing more water while exercising at the time of fasting is always recom- mended.

•**Keeping up the electrolytes:** It is very important to keep up your electrolytes at

the time of working out. You can try out coconut water for replenishing the electrolytes. Moreover, it is very low in calorie count and also tastes good. Opting for energy drinks such as Gatorade is not recommended as they come with high sugar content. So, it is better to avoid them as much as possible.

•**Keeping the duration and intensity low:** If you try to push your
 body too hard
from the very beginning, it might result in dizziness and fatigue. If you
cannot take up the load, just take a break. There is no need to be forceful
on your body. You need to properly listen to your body if you want to
yield the best re- sults. Try to reduce the duration of your workout
session during the first few weeks.

•**Considering the fast type:** The type of fast that you are performin
g has a lot to
do with your workout session. For instance, if you are practicing an
inter- mittent fast for 24 hours, you need to keep the intensity of your
exercise as low as possible. If you are doing 16/8 fast, you can opt for
the hardcore exer- cises as you can rest your body during the 16 hours
window.

Various Types of Exercises

The type of workout that you pick up for losing weight has a lot to do
with the end results. Also, you need to choose something that you really
enjoy so that you can stick to it as your daily routine.

•**Aerobics:** Despite the type of workout program that you implement
in your
routine, it is of utter importance that you include some sort of
cardiovascular or aerobic exercise in your routine. It can help in getting
the rate of your heart up and can also pump up your blood. You can
start with jogging, walking, cy- cling, dancing, or swimming. You can
also opt for any kind of fitness ma- chines such as a stair stepper,
treadmill, and others.

•**Weight training:** The biggest advantage that comes along with wei
ght training
is that, besides losing fast, you can also build up your muscles. When
you have more muscles, you can burn calories much more easily. You
need to work on all the major groups of muscles 3 times a week. The
major muscle groups include back, abs, calves, chest, biceps, triceps,
traps, shoulders, forearms, hamstrings, and quads.

Before Starting With Your Exercise Program If you are thinking about exercising while fasting, it is always recommended to talk to your doctor at first. If you are having certain conditions such as diabetes, lung disease, heart disease, arthritis, and kidney disease, make sure that you go through a proper checkup right before starting with the program. As you start with the pro- gram, try to notice the signals that your body is giving out. Try to push yourself a bit every day to improve your level of fitness. Do not just jump into some sort of hardcore exercise from the first day.

CHAPTER 9: HOW TO MANAGE MENOPAUSE

The phase of menopause starts from the age of the late 40s or from the early 50s for the majority of women. Menopause generally lasts for some years. But, the time period of menopause is not at all smooth. It has been found that almost 63% of women go through the symptoms that are related to menopause. The symptoms of menopause are varying in nature. Let's have a look at some of the most common symptoms of menopause.

•**Irregular periods:** The early onset of menopause can be identified by periods
at irregular intervals.

•**Dryness:** Women might suffer from vaginal dryness.

•**Night sweats:** Sudden sweating at nighttime.

•**Mood swings:** This is a very common symptom that includes chang ing of
mood from good to bad and again from bad to good.

•**Gain in body weight:** There might be a sudden increase in overall body
weight. Symptoms, such as changes in the cycle of menstruation vary from women to women. Generally, you will be experiencing some irregular nature of periods right before they tend to end. The skipping of periods at the time of menopause is very common. The cycle of menstruation might skip one month and then return again, or might skip several months and then begin with normal monthly cycles after a few months. The cycle of periods will also tend to be shorter than usual. Also, women who are going through menopause have higher chances of developing var- ious diseases such as diabetes, heart disease, obesity along with osteoporosis.

Eating Food Items Rich In Vitamin D And Calcium

During menopause, hormonal changes take place. This might result in the weak- ening of the bones. Thus, it can also increase the risk of developing osteoporosis. Vitamin D and calcium are often linked with good health of bones. So, you are re- quired to include enough of all these nutrients within your daily diet. Proper intake of Vitamin D in women who are going through menopause is also linked with a lesser risk of any kind of hip fractures because of the weak nature of the bones. You can find various food items that are rich in calcium content such as milk, cheese, and yogurt. Fresh green vegetables such as spinach, kale, and collard greens come with high quantities of calcium. You can get the same from beans, sardines, beans, and various other food items. You can also opt for calcium- fortified food items such as fruit juice, alternatives of milk, and certain types of cereals. Sunlight is regarded as the primary source of Vitamin D as it can be produced by our skin when it gets exposed to sunlight. But, with growing age, the capability of the skin for producing Vitamin D from sunlight tends to decrease. In case you do not like being in the sunlight for a long time, you can opt for Vitamin D supple- ments and various food items that are rich in Vitamin D content. You can have oily fish, cod liver oil, eggs, and Vitamin D fortified food items. So, for dealing with weak bones at the time of menopause, having a proper amount of Vitamin D and calcium in your diet is very important.

Maintaining And Achieving Healthy Body Weight

A very common symptom at the time of menopause is weight gain. This generally results from changes in hormones, lifestyle, genetics, and aging. When you an gain excessive amount of body fat, specifically around your waist, it increases the risk of developing various diseases like diabetes and heart disease. The symptoms of menopause might also get affected because of excessive body weight. It has been found that women who are able to shed almost 10% - 15% of their body weight at the time of menopause can easily eliminate the chances of having night sweat and hot flashes. So, it is very important to maintain your body weight for dealing with the various symptoms of menopause. **Consuming Lots Of Veggies And Fruits** When you have a diet that is rich in veggies and fruits, you can easily prevent var- ious symptoms of menopause. Vegetables and fruits come with low-calorie count and can help you in feeling full easily. So, it can be said that vegetables and fruits are great for losing weight and maintenance of the same. Fruits and vegetables can also help in dealing with various types of heart diseases. Having fruits and vegeta- bles daily is important especially after menopause as the risk of developing heart disease also tends to increase. This is probably because of the various factors like gain in weight, age, or reduced levels of estrogen. Also, having fruits and veggies can help in dealing with the loss of bones.

Avoiding Trigger Foods

There are certain types of food items that can effectively trigger the symptoms of menopause such as night sweats, mood swings, and hot flashes. They are most likely to trigger the symptoms when consumed at night. Some of the most com- mon triggers include alcohol, spicy and sugary food items, and caffeine. You can try to keep a diary of symptoms. If you think that some particular food item is trig- gering your symptoms of menopause, you can reduce the consumption of such food items or completely avoid them.

Exercising Regularly

Although there is not an adequate amount of evidence for supporting that

exercising can help in dealing with night sweats and hot flashes. But, it can help in dealing with other problems. It helps in improving your metabolism and energy, re- sults in healthier bones and joints, better nature of sleep, and reduced stress. One study found out that regular exercising for about 3 hours every week for one com- plete year can help in improving the mental and physical health along with the overall life quality of menopausal women. It can also help in preventing various diseases such as heart disease, cancer, type 2 diabetes, high blood pressure, stroke, osteoporosis, and obesity.

Eating Food Items Rich In Phytoestrogens

Phytoestrogens are the plant compounds that occur naturally and can mimic the overall effects of estrogen in our bodies. Thus, they can help in balancing all the hormones. High intake of this compound in the Asian countries like Japan is re- garded as the primary reason why women going through menopause in such places experience hot flashes rarely. There are various foods that are rich in phytoe- strogens such as tofu, soybeans, tempeh, linseeds, flaxseeds, beans, and sesame seeds. But, the overall content of phytoestrogens in the food items depends on the methods of processing. It has been that diets that are high in soy can help in reducing the levels of cholesterol, blood pressure, reduced severity of the symp- toms of menopause such as night sweats and hot flashes among all those women who are undergoing menopause. **Drinking Enough Water** Women are very likely to experience dryness at the time of menopause. This is mainly because of the decrease in the levels of estrogen. For dealing with such symptoms, you can drink around 10-12 glasses of water every day. It also helps in reducing the feeling of bloating that can result because of the hormonal changes.

Additionally, water helps in dealing with weight gain and also aids in the loss of weight by making you feel full. Water can also increase the metabolism of your body. Drinking around 500ml of water about half an hour before having your meal can help you in consuming 14% fewer calories while having the meal.

Reducing Processed Foods And Refined Sugar

When you have a diet plan which is high in sugar and refined carbs, it can result in sharp dips and rises in the level of blood sugar and thus making you feel irritable and tired. In fact, it has been found that meals that are very high in refined carbs content can readily increase the overall risk of developing depression in women who just finished off with their menopause. Also, diets that are full of processed foods can affect the health of your bones. So, for better health of the bones, it is necessary to keep out processed foods and refined sugar from your daily diet.

Not Skipping Meals

It is very important to have regular meals as you are going through the period of menopause. When you indulge in irregular eating patterns, it can worsen certain symptoms of menopause and can also hinder all the efforts of weight loss. It is essential to keep all your nutritional requirements on point while going through menopause.

Eating Foods Rich In Protein

Regularly having protein-rich foods can help in the prevention of losing all the lean muscle that generally results because of aging. It has been found from a study that consuming protein all throughout the day can slow down the loss of muscles that result from aging. Also, besides maintaining lean muscle mass, protein-rich foods also help in losing weight as they help on making you feel full and also increase the total calories which are burnt. You can get enough protein from food items such as fish, meat, eggs, dairy, nuts, and legumes.

Dealing With Night Sweats

You can opt for various strategies for dealing with night sweats. Try to dress in light clothes at night. Opt for layered bedding so that it gets easier for you to remove them at night. Sleep by keeping an electric fan beside you. Try to drink cool water all throughout the course of the night at regular intervals. You can keep an ice pack right under your pillow so that you can turn over the pil- low at times for making sure that your head is resting on the cool surface all the time.

Practicing Techniques Of Relaxation

You can start with techniques of relaxation such as paced breathing, deep breath- ing, massage, progressive relaxation of muscles, and guided imagery for helping yourself with the various symptoms of menopause. You need to stay relaxed for controlling night sweats and hot flashes.

Quit Smoking

Smoking can readily increase the risks of developing stroke, heart disease, cancer, osteoporosis, and several other health-related problems. Moreover, it can readily increase the severity of hot flashes and night sweats. Also, smoking can bring in the early onset of menopause.

Dealing With Urinary Problems

Many women develop urinary and bladder problems at the time of menopause. This is mainly because of the lower levels of estrogen that results in weakening of the urethra. Some women might even find it very difficult to hold their urine for a long time without going to the bathroom. This is known as urinary urge incon- tinence. There are also high chances of urine leaking when you cough, laugh or sneeze. This is known as urinary stress incontinence. For dealing with all these, you need to reduce or avoid having caffeine, taking medication, physical therapy, or even surgery, depending on the condition. You can also consult your doctor if the condition worsens.

Reducing Anxiety And Depression

At the time of menopause, the chances of developing anxiety and depression in- crease. This is mainly caused because of hormonal changes. You might go through feelings of sadness as changes occur in your body. Also, anxiety and depression can worsen the symptoms of menopause. You need to limit the consumption of alcohol as it can readily result in depression. Also, getting enough sleep can help.

Dealing With Mood Swings

A very common symptom of menopause is mood swings. Women might feel irri- tated or disturbed with even the smallest things. You need to keep yourself active to help deal with mood swings. If you are not active enough, try finding out ways in which you can be active. Also, do not try to take excessive duties at once. Look out for the positive ways in which you can ease your symptoms of stress.

When To See A Doctor

If the symptoms of menopause are bothering you, try consulting with your doctor. While talking about your problems make sure to discuss all the symptoms that you are facing and also the extent of the same. Also, talk with the doctor if you have undergone any kind of treatment for dealing with the symptoms of menopause be- fore.

CONCLUSION

The good thing about Intermittent fasting is that it is a very straight forward and easy to follow a diet that will change your life for the better. All the useful techniques and mistakes to avoid when fasting can help with going through the diet without any hitches.

As we have seen, intermittent fasting is extremely beneficial for the body, especially health-wise. Healthy individuals should do intermittent fasting at least once to get all the benefits that come with intermittent fasting. You can easily make intermittent fasting part of your day to day life. If you find that you keep failing, all you need to do is reduce your fasting window and keep going.

Although it is a new way of looking at dieting and nutrition there are some clear health benefits. Further testing on human beings needs to be investigated and researched before we can say there are substantial long-term effects of intermittent fasting, but so far the signs are good. Just make sure you don't fall for the potential risks and you are clear why you are doing it and stay in control of your diet.

Printed by Libri Plureos GmbH in Hamburg,
Germany